Dermatologic Surgery with Radiofrequency

Art of Successful Practice

Dermatologic Surgery with Radiofrequency

Art of Successful Practice

Bipin Deshpande

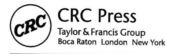

CRC Press
Taylor & Francis Group
Boca Raton London New York

CRC Press is an imprint of the
Taylor & Francis Group, an **informa** business

CRC Press
Taylor & Francis Group
6000 Broken Sound Parkway NW, Suite 300
Boca Raton, FL 33487-2742

First issued in paperback 2020

ISBN-13: 978-0-367-57167-2 (pbk)
ISBN-13: 978-1-138-30114-6 (hbk)

Library of Congress Cataloging-in-Publication Data

Names: Deshpande, Bipin, author.
Title: Dermatologic surgery with radiofrequency : art of successful practice / Bipin Deshpande.
Description: Boca Raton, FL : CRC Press/Taylor & Francis Group, 2018. | Includes bibliographical references and index.
Identifiers: LCCN 2017057558| ISBN 9781138301146 (hardback : alk. paper) | ISBN 9780203732182 (ebook : alk. paper)
Subjects: | MESH: Dermatologic Surgical Procedures--methods | Pulsed Radiofrequency Treatment--methods | Ambulatory Surgical Procedures--methods
Classification: LCC RD655 | NLM WR 670 | DDC 617.4/77--dc23
LC record available at https://lccn.loc.gov/2017057558

Visit the Taylor & Francis Web site at
http://www.taylorandfrancis.com

and the CRC Press Web site atW
http://www.crcpress.com

I dedicate this book to the "inspiring memories" of my late father Shri Bhaskar Shripad Deshpande, who had always inspired me throughout my childhood and career to be a compassionate and helpful medical practitioner.

Bipin Deshpande

Contents

Foreword

In the early 1980s, CO_2 lasers were adopted by dermatologic surgeons and were widely featured in medical journal articles. A few years later, I had the privilege of participating in a formal debate held as a plenary session at the scientific meeting of the American Society for Dermatologic Surgery. In the debate, an expert in CO_2 laser surgery (Dr. Philip Bailin) and I, representing radiosurgery (then "electrosurgery"), were given the opportunity to convince the audience as to which modality was superior. At the conclusion of this session, attendees voted and were found to favor electrosurgery over laser, by a margin of 7 to 1! Factors relating to cost, ease of training, mobility of the equipment, and versatility were all determinants of that decision. These positive attributes of radiosurgery remain today.

I have adopted many new technologies, including laser, over the years, but radiofrequency remains an irreplaceable modality in my cosmetic dermatologic surgery practice. Although radiosurgery is performed thousands of times around the globe each day, it has been many years since a new text highlighting its use has appeared. Despite the emergence of many modern energy-based technologies, utilizing a variety of laser, ultrasonic, and other concussive and thermal formats, radiofrequency remains a readily available and inexpensive solution to many dermatologic surgical needs, particularly in less developed countries.

Dr. Bipin Deshpande has been a devoted practitioner and educator on this subject for nearly two decades, and his book, *Dermatologic Surgery with Radiofrequency*, is the culmination of his explorations and the insights that he has garnered. The monograph not only provides detailed treatment information but, in addition, illustrates how radiofrequency fits into the overall setting of dermatologic surgery. Moreover, the reader has an opportunity to explore and hone new skills by using the included practice sessions. I applaud Dr. Deshpande for his tireless efforts to keep the importance of radiofrequency alive in the next generation of practitioners.

Sheldon V. Pollack, MD
Associate Professor of Medicine (Dermatology)
University of Toronto

Preface

Medical practice is an art that is learned through experience built up over decades of hard work. This can never be taught in medical colleges. Art has no boundaries or limits, so much so that any good and learned practitioner not only can be a successful practitioner, but with devotion and effort can specialize in a novel field.

I remember a practicing anesthesiologist in India who after 10 years began specializing in the field of dermatologic surgery and cosmetic dermatology. He successfully transformed himself into an (an)aesthetic practitioner.

I started my practice as a family physician in the metropolitan city of Pune, India, in 1988. I had done my specialization in dermatology but only practiced it occasionally. I always like to be off the beaten track, and even in family practice I presented many novel studies at local conferences. Simultaneously, I studied light and its effects on skin (photobiomodulation) way back in 1996 and am still doing these treatments. I have presented many studies on photobiomodulation at various national and international conferences.

I find the field of dermatology very challenging; many skin diseases have recurrences, which can be frustrating to patients as well as doctors. The therapy angle is very narrow and with side effects. Managing skin diseases with limited medicines is an art. After years of managing the same patients with the same problems or new patients with the same problems, when one day you experience the "one shot treatment" of dermatologic surgery where a patient is cleared of his or her skin problem, it is really like a refreshing drink after toiling in the hot sun.

Radiofrequency surgery was to me a "refreshing drink." It refreshed me so much when I experienced its results that it became my passion. The happiness that came along with the successful results and the great patient satisfaction because of no recurrence was itself a great inspiration to explore and do more.

I introduced radiofrequency surgery in Indian dermatology at the National Dermatology Conference in 2000. Since then, radiofrequency surgery has received an overwhelming response in all dermatology societies. I have spoken on many national and international podiums, conducted teaching workshops, and written many articles.

Believe me, I have never marketed my services. My patients are my best walking and talking advertisements.

Many doctors from faculties other than dermatology have shown great interest in radiofrequency surgery. Some have learned from me, but there are many more who would still like to learn the technique. For them and purely clinical dermatologists and all the new budding dermatologists, this book will be of great assistance not only as a guide but as a step-by-step learning book to practice radiofrequency surgery at their bests in their own clinics or offices.

There was no valuable publication on the use of radiofrequency surgery in dermatologic surgery for more than a decade. There are numerous publications on lasers and radiofrequency for skin tightening and body contouring, as well as fractional radiofrequency for acne scars. While conducting workshops, the attending doctors expressed the need of a publication on uses of radiofrequency for dermatologic surgery. Hence, I have made an effort to compile my data and personal experiences to write this book.

I have written this book as a "storybook" that slowly and steadily unravels the basic as well as the "gems and jewels" of radiofrequency surgery. I have tried to use simple language to cover almost all aspects of the surgery required for clinic-based practice. I have also made it very practical with a large collection of my case study photos and schematic illustrations. Most of the after photos are given to show the immediate postoperative appearance of wound, which can result in least or negligible scarring. It is for the readers to understand that if they can achieve such a postoperative wound on the operating table, they are assured a best result.

The book's final chapter takes readers to an imaginary world but emphasizes the importance of scientific knowledge and the limits of technology.

My sincere and best wishes to you!

Acknowledgments

It was my real dream to write a book on radiofrequency surgery since the time I started in the field. It has been a very interesting 18 years and it is now a passion. All these tireless years, I have been through practical research of my own and education with the help of thousands of photographs and numerous lectures and workshops for the budding and already practicing dermatologists. Over this period there have been many good people who have helped me with kind advice without expecting any returns.

I must thank Dr. Jon Garito, former president of Ellman International Inc., New York, for his very friendly advice and help in the initial period.

I thank Dr. Dileep Mane, chairman cum managing director, Noble Hospital, Pune, India, for his kind help in allowing me to organize so many radiofrequency surgery teaching workshops.

A special word of thanks and my love and gratitude for my wife, Anjali, and son, Dr. Ruchir, who have very patiently supported me and inspired me throughout these tireless 18 years always with a smile. It is their sacrifice that has helped me to rise to such a height on this academic front.

I express my love and special gratitude to my mother, Sushanta, who was always a driving force to me in my early childhood, without which I would never have seen these days.

Finally, I thank Mr. Bharat Ketkar, a professional artist who has done such wonderful line drawings and illustrations for my book.

Author

Dr. Bipin Deshpande, MBBS, DVD, FAAD, has been a practicing dermatologist for 29 years. He is the head of the Department of Cosmetology at Noble Hospital, a leading hospital in Pune, India. He attended St. Vincent's High School and B. J. Medical College, Pune.

Dr. Deshpande has been an International Fellow of the American Academy of Dermatology for 12 years. He is also a life member of the Indian Association of Dermatologists, Venereologists and Leprologists; Cosmetic Dermatology Society of India; and Indian Medical Association.

He specializes in cosmetic dermatology, dermatologic surgery, and laser therapy. He has been a pioneer in India in the fields of radiofrequency surgery and photobiomodulation, and he introduced radiofrequency surgery in Indian dermatology in 2000 at the National Dermatology Conference. He also introduced photobiomodulation with the help of the case study article "Diabetic Ulcer Treated by BioBeam 660 Phototherapy" in the *Indian Journal of Dermatology, Venereology and Leprology* in 1996.

He has presented more than 40 original research papers at national dermatology conferences and national cutaneous surgery conferences. He has also presented more than 30 original research papers at various international dermatology conferences including the World Congress of Dermatology, American Academy of Dermatology, World Congress of Family Physicians, International League of Dermatology with Egyptian Women's Dermatology Society joint conference, DASIL (Dermatologic and Aesthetic Surgery International League), and IMCAS (Internal Master Course on Aging Skin).

He has conducted more than 50 teaching workshops in India for radiofrequency surgery and one workshop in Cairo, Egypt. He has been a guest speaker at many local, regional, and national conferences.

His chapter contributions include "Radiofrequency Surgery: Ablative and Non-Ablative" in the *Manual of Cosmetic Dermatology and Surgery* published in 2009, and "Radiofrequency and Electrocautery" in the book *Procedures in Dermatosurgery: Step by Step Approach* to be published in early 2018.

He was conferred in *Who's Who in Medicine and Healthcare* in 2007 and 2009, *Who's Who in Asia* in 2007, and *Who's Who in World* in 2008 by *Marquis Who's Who*.

Deshpande has an Indian patent for designing an instrument for facial scar management.

Introduction

Dermatologic surgery, or cutaneous surgery, is an ever-expanding and sought after field. The ever-increasing demand for surgery in dermatology is not the only reason for it. There is a growing demand for dermatologic surgery from many fields of medicine, including general surgery, otorhinolaryngology, ophthalmology, plastic and reconstructive surgery, and family practice. Dermatologic surgery was and is still being performed quite commonly using the "gold standard" scalpel or the favorite modalities of contemporary clinical dermatologists like electrocautery and cryosurgery.

Dermatologic surgery generally fits into the category of minor surgery. For decades general practitioners or family physicians performed these surgeries in their small setups. Dermatologic surgery in family practice started dwindling in the last three decades as more specialized surgical care became available with advanced technology. Technological advances and availability of different medical specialties even made family practice a specialty of its own. The dermatologic surgery also became specialized with the development of electrosurgery, radiofrequency surgery, and lasers. The development of punches facilitated doing skin biopsy.

Dermatologic surgery involves surgery related to all skin diseases for diagnostic and therapeutic purposes. Skin diseases include cutaneous, venereal, and leprologic diseases.

Decades earlier, before the advent of electrosurgery and lasers, lesions were removed using the modalities of a scalpel, hyfrecator, electrocautery, cryosurgery, or chemical cautery. Here, the final result involved complete removal of lesion where the residual scar hardly mattered.

In the modern era, there is an additional demand from patients due to cosmetic concern of facial skin and other body parts. This has expanded the scope of dermatologic surgery to the present stage where it involves giving more specialized surgical services to reduce the operative time and postoperative downtime as well as resulting in minimum complications and negligible residual scarring.

In the early 20th century the methods of dermatologic surgery were very crude. Some of these small skin surgeries were performed by licensed medical practitioners. But, I recall that in rural or semiurban areas such surgical work was carried out by unlicensed practitioners or quacks with complications. Though the scalpel and cryosurgery or electrocautery were used, most of the skin lesions on bodily skin and genitalia were removed leaving obvious scarring or suture marks (Figures 1.1 and 1.2). These were accepted without prejudice or mistrust.

The better knowledge and applications of electric current, electromagnetism, laser physics and their connections as well as applications on the biological tissues made huge progress in the later part of the 20th century. The development of good quality electrosurgery equipment dates back to 1926 and is credited to Harvard physicist William Bovie. This was preceded by many earlier experiments to develop equipment using electric current for skin surgery. The Bovie electrosurgery equipment was reasonably complete comprising of both cutting and coagulation currents. This was further improvised to include more facilities for better removal of superficial as well as deep lesions. Thus the newer equipment using higher frequencies allowed electrosection, electrocoagulation, electrodesiccation, and fulguration, which led to more precise and effective dermatologic surgery. Lasers, which became available after 1960, have been a favorite of modern-day dermatologists.

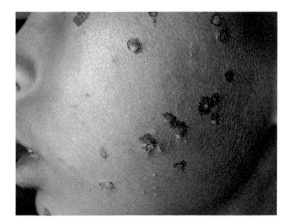

Figure 1.1 Postchemical cautery scabs and burnt skin.

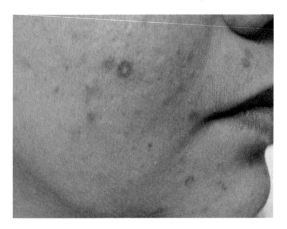

Figure 1.2 Postelectrocautery scars.

The educational curriculum of dermatology at many institutions has yet to include modern electrosurgery and lasers. In fact, there is a need to update the educational curriculum to include these and modern radiofrequency surgery universally. Because of this drawback, dermatologists were hardly well equipped to surgically deal with skin lesions. This lack of confidence among dermatologists led to many skin lesions being tackled by surgeon colleagues. There was also a lack of awareness among the general public as to the best surgical treatment for skin lesions.

Dermatologic surgical care given by surgeons from any faculty, whether general surgery or others, appeared to lack in the dexterity compared to their dermatology colleagues. This lack is likely due to either use of their favorite scalpel or surgical diathermy or due to lack of awareness of the

histopathology of the concerned dermatological lesions. The advantage dermatologists have in doing dermatologic surgery is that they are well aware of the histopathology of the concerned skin lesions. They know the best level to reach in order for complete removal with minimal or no scarring.

The dermatologic surgery described in this book is confined to the minor operating theater or office surgery, which is performed in a clinic-based setup. While performing such procedures, one must be perfectly clear in the scope and limitations of them. One must be fully confident in performing these procedures totally in the office with or without the help of staff. One must also be absolutely clear with the criteria of performing dermatologic surgical procedures in the hospital operation theater. Although these criteria may vary between professionals, the overall accepted ones are mentioned in Table 1.1.

Office dermatologic surgery has advantages and disadvantages, which are mentioned in Tables 1.2 and 1.3. Office dermatologic surgery can be

Table 1.1 Criteria for doing hospital-based dermatologic surgery

- Pediatric patients under 6 years of age
- Geriatric patients: No age limit, but patients have cardiac or other major risk factors
- Patients with bleeding disorders
- Patients with lesions that are likely to bleed significantly during surgery
- Patients with lesions close to sensitive areas of body such as the eyes, inside nostrils, or in the oral cavity
- Very anxious and noncooperative patients
- Immunocompromised patients
- Cancer patients
- Patients with HIV and HBV infection

Table 1.2 Advantages of office dermatologic surgery

- Patient is more comfortable
- Less time-consuming
- Easy to plan and perform
- Minimum investigations
- Fewer restrictions
- Rapid biopsy
- Financial saving
- Instant surgical treatment possible

Table 1.3 Disadvantages of office dermatologic surgery

- All skin lesions cannot be tackled effectively
- Limitation of space, disinfection facilities
- Limitations of surgical time
- Likely to miss serious pathology
- Limitations of anesthesia (general anesthesia cannot be given)
- Lack of sufficient staff
- Fear of medicolegal implications if any serious complications occur

performed effectively using a scalpel, electrocautery, cryosurgery, electrosurgery, radiofrequency surgery, or lasers. I used the first three modalities early in my career. Once I started using radiofrequency surgery I found that it had potential to replace not only all the earlier ones but also could be a better alternative to ablative lasers.

A survey was conducted among dermatologists (young and budding as well as those having 10 years or more experience) to find the choice of modality for dermatologic surgery. The survey was done using a small, easy-to-complete questionnaire circulated in semiurban areas and metropolitan cities in India. The survey was sent to 100 dermatologists having practice experience between 4 and 20 years. Eighty-five dermatologists completed the survey. The first part of the survey contained questions related to dermatologic surgery in practice and the second part contained questions related to radiofrequency surgery in practice. The results of this survey revealed that a majority of dermatologists preferred using

radiofrequency surgery for office dermatologic surgery.

The results of the first part of the survey are as follows:

- All dermatologists performed dermatologic surgery.
- Most (more than 80%) had electrocautery and radiofrequency surgery.
- Only a few (less than 20%) had all modalities of electrocautery, scalpel, cryosurgery, lasers and radiofrequency surgery.
- Most (more than 80%) agree that 10% to 25% of practice is contributed by dermatologic surgery; only few have less than 10% or more than 25%.
- All agree that "dermatologic surgery is an indispensable part of dermatology practice" today.

The results of the second part of the survey are given in Chapter 5.

Office dermatologic surgery has the clear advantage of an "instant organization within practice." This makes it possible to make immediate or on-the-spot decisions for quick consultation and surgery. This is time-saving for patients and quick revenue-building for doctors. The clinic or office should be predesigned or modified to suit this advantage. Additional staff or assistant help should be planned for proper implementation of this service. It is always possible for any medical professional, whether dermatologist or surgeon from any faculty, to give this service during routine consulting practice hours as time-gap adjustments or preplanned hours on particular days of the week.

Office dermatologic surgery

Clinic-based dermatologic surgery is performed in the office or clinic of a clinician. Any clinician having reasonable knowledge and confidence can perform the surgery. Any clinician who has a routine clinical practice as a physician can later modify his or her practice to perform dermatologic surgery after acquiring sufficient knowledge and skills. Here, my advice is to have full inclination and intention to do so.

A clinician or practitioner from any faculty of medicine can develop and establish an office dermatologic surgery. Following are some of my suggestions before developing this practice:

- Total inclination and devotion
- Sufficient space in clinic to devote to this activity
- Minimum requirements of minor operating theater
- Quiet and clean surroundings
- Sufficient operating skills
- Reasonably trained staff
- Investment in reasonably good and advanced surgical technology considering the array of various dermatological conditions one needs to deal with

I will next expand on these suggestions.

Total inclination and devotion. Dermatologic surgery on facial or bodily skin requires good understanding of the histopathology of the relevant skin lesions to be tackled. In today's world, cosmesis is of primary concern, hence all such surgeries need to be given sufficient time and care for best results. Best results will be delivered only with total inclination and devotion. One should avoid any interruption or disturbance of phone calls or other activities of the clinic.

Sufficient space in clinic. Office-based dermatologic surgery requires a minimum of 140 square feet floor area. It is always desirable to have a separate room for this area rather than assigning a small cubicle in a large consulting room.

Minimum requirements of minor operating theater.[1] The room delegated for dermatologic surgery should be properly designed and equipped for the job (Figure 2.1). The requirements are described in brief next:

- Room color should be light or pale white/yellow for good illumination.
- Flooring can be of light-colored tiles or carpet (nonslippery).
- LED tube lights are best for good illumination.
- Electrical fixtures in the form of ceiling and wall-mounted fans, exhaust fans, air conditioner, sufficient sockets for connecting different equipment, and extension boards.
- Inverter with sufficient battery backup for covering at least 3 hours in case of unexpected electricity failure.
- An operating magnifying lens with a circular tube light fitted around the lens, which is sufficient for any surgeries to be performed in the clinic (Figure 2.2). It has the advantage of giving a magnified view for clean and clear dissection as well as good cosmesis.
- Surgical trolleys (one or two) for keeping surgical equipment, syringes, dressing material, bandages, paper tapes, tissue papers, surface and local anesthetics, emergency medicine, sphygmomanometer, alcohol-based antiseptic, povidone-iodine, normal saline, sterilized cotton, forceps (plain, toothed, and artery), kidney trays, and formal saline-filled plain bulbs for biopsy materials (Figure 2.3).

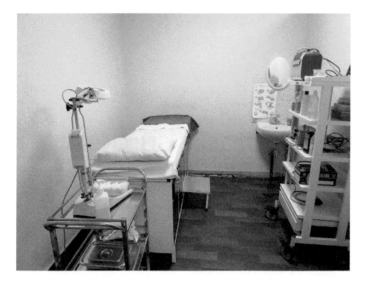

Figure 2.1 Minor operating theater (office dermatologic surgery), Noble Hospital, Pune, India.

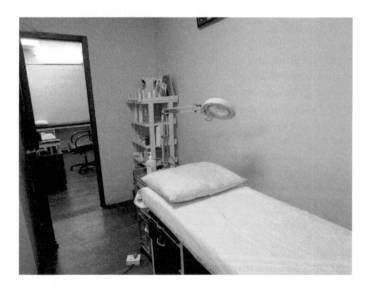

Figure 2.2 Operating bed with magnifying lens.

- Washbasin and two waste bins (one for surgery-related materials and the second for routine waste).
- Wall-mounted mirror and hand-held mirror (for patient to use postsurgery).
- Music player with speakers for playing soft, soothing music in the background for relieving anxiety of patients thus creating a relaxing environment in the operating room.

Quiet and clean surroundings. An office for dermatologic surgery needs a clean dust-free environment and quiet surroundings for efficient surgical procedures (Figure 2.4).

Sufficient operating skills. All clinicians, dermatologists or otherwise, ought to acquire sufficient operating skills with their preferred modality before going into full-fledged dermatologic surgery. They must always be up to date and try to employ the latest techniques with minimum downtime and negligible scarring.

Reasonably trained staff. A staff is usually preferred to assist during office dermatologic surgery. An effort must be made to train such a

parameters of the operating equipment. The staff should also be trained for handling situations of vasovagal shock or helping during emergencies. A close relative of the patient can be allowed to sit inside the operating room to further boost the confidence of the patient as well as relieve anxiety of the relative in the case of a child, the elderly, or pregnant woman.

Investment in good, effective surgical technology. A judicious investment in the best surgical technology will always give unlimited returns in the form of name, fame, and monetary returns. This decision is very critical, as such investment has to be done considering one's budget, aim of surgical practice, easy operability, best results, space occupancy, maintenance, and recurring costs.

It is much easier to learn radiofrequency surgery though it requires proper training to understand the functioning of this technique. All details regarding this are covered at length in the relevant chapters in the later part of this book. In fact, any clinician or surgeon using other surgical modalities can also specialize in the use of radiofrequency surgery for dermatologic surgery. Switchover tips are explained in detail later.

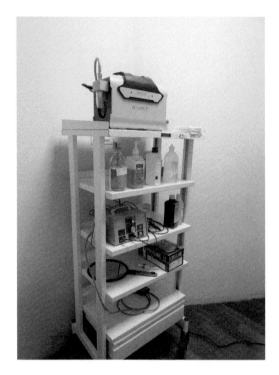

Figure 2.3 Surgical trolley containing radiofrequency equipment and other requisites for office surgery.

staff to assist while giving local anesthetic injection and calming patients if they are panicky. The staff should also help in preparing patients for minor surgery, helping with instruments during surgery, and modifying the power or other

REFERENCE

1. Brown JS. Minor operating theater, In: *Minor Surgery: A Text and Atlas*, 4th edition, London, Arnold Publishers, 2000.

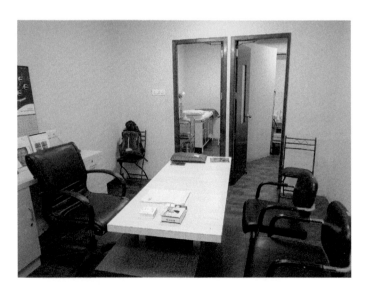

Figure 2.4 Consulting room with adjoining operating theater and laser room.

3

Prerequisites of office dermatologic surgery

Prerequisites of office dermatologic surgery done using any surgical modality remain the same. This chapter considers more issues that are an integral part of this surgery.

PREOPERATIVE CLINICAL ASSESSMENT

All patients posted for dermatologic surgery need to be counseled about the procedure. The counseling may take 15 to 30 minutes. The assessment centers upon two main concerns: (1) the ideal patient and (2) frequently asked questions and patient counseling.

The ideal patient

The patient is the center of the whole show of office dermatologic surgery. The patient posted for surgery must be in a stable mental state. He or she should also be fully prepared for the planned surgery, its final result, and its possible side effects and shortcomings. All doubts and fears about surgery or its postoperative cosmesis must be totally cleared from the patient's mind. The patient should not have unrealistic expectations.

Frequently asked questions and patient counseling

All patients, whether stable or anxious, have basic questions they will ask before any surgery, including:

- How much pain during and postsurgery?
- Will surgery fully clear the concerned problem?

- Will surgery worsen my facial appearance (in case of facial lesion)?
- How much time is needed for full recovery?
- Will there be a need for me to take leave from work for recovery?
- Will there be any scars?

These frequently asked questions and many more should be satisfactorily answered and all other doubts of the patient must be effectively cleared through a very candid and clear discussion. This positive counseling should lead to boosting the patient's confidence and building of a good relationship of mutual trust between patient and surgeon.

THE IDEAL DERMATOLOGIC SURGEON

All dermatologic surgeons are expected to possess certain qualities, including the following:

- Depth of knowledge and understanding of the skin lesions to be removed
- Adequate training and experience to handle such cases
- Technical aptitude and dexterity to use radiofrequency surgery to deliver the best results
- Adequate patience to understand patient's expectations and work systematically to achieve promised results
- Never overpromise results, always be patient during surgery using radiofrequency, and never be overzealous in order to avoid complications

STAFF OR ASSISTANTS

Dermatologic surgery usually requires only one to two assistants. Generally, a single assistant is good enough for radiofrequency surgery. An assistant helps with preoperative preparation of the patient and making all requirements ready beforehand, including preoperative sterilization and minimum required documentation. They can also assist with simple tasks during the procedure like holding forceps, during hemorrhage, alleviating fears of anxious patients, and postoperative dressing. An assistant need not be a paramedic (though a trained nurse always makes a difference) but should be stable minded and have good endurance. Good experience is a must for such a job. Preoperative and postoperative documentation, histopathology specimen handling, and record keeping should be responsibly carried out by an assistant. The assistant staff does not need to be fully scrubbed and wearing sterile gloves during operation unless their active participation is required.

ROLE OF PATIENT'S ACCOMPANIMENT

Any patient who is posted for dermatologic surgery is always a bit uncomfortable, anxious, or apprehensive before start of the surgical procedure. I always allow the patient's accompaniment (spouse, friend, parent, guardian) inside the operating room to alleviate this feeling. The patient is always more comfortable having the accompanying person close inside the operating room than without, because the patient is in an unfamiliar environment during the procedure. The accompanying person is not required to be scrubbed; they can just wear the footwear meant for an operating room and sit at a specified comfortable distance in the room. Their presence makes the operating environment more relaxed. In fact, even the accompanying person feels more comfortable than sitting outside waiting anxiously. I have seen that this simple allowance reflects a good gesture on the part of the surgeon as far as confidence and transparency is concerned. However, I always take precaution not to allow any qualmy accompanying person, for example, someone who cannot stand the sight of blood or seeing the patient being injected or operated upon, who may spoil the situation.

PREOPERATIVE STERILIZATION

Sterilization of all materials used for office surgery should be carried out with the authentic methods of sterilization such as the autoclave or hot air ovens. The materials include all the instruments used in operation, that is, the forceps, needle holders, scalpels, blades, electrodes, and other relevant tools. If any office surgeries are to be performed with the radiofrequency method on an urgent basis, I steam-sterilize the electrodes.

SENSITIVITY TESTING

Lignocaine sensitivity, though very low (<1%), should be included in the protocol for all patients for safety purposes. I have encountered sensitivity to topical surface anesthetic cream in my practice, though very rarely.

INTRAOPERATIVE REQUIREMENTS

All operations are planned beforehand. The planning includes the selection of instrument, electrodes, good illumination, and magnifying lens. Patient skin preparation is always done with standard protocol using povidone-iodine followed by absolute alcohol. Normal saline, sterilized gauze pieces, cotton balls, dressing materials, paper tape, and postoperative soothing gels (for patients treated with electrodessication) are also part of these requirements. A hand mirror is essential for all patients to see themselves immediately after office surgery done on the face.

POSTOPERATIVE CARE

All patients in office surgery are conscious and aware of all the events taking place during surgery. Postoperative care consists of dressings and advice to be followed regarding medicines, soap use during baths, and other relevant matters. Follow-up visits are advised as well. Specific care pertaining to radiofrequency surgery is covered later.

4

Selection of surgical modality

Dermatologic surgical procedures are performed most commonly in an office. As I have said earlier, this surgery fits into the category of minor surgery. There are various modalities used in surgery from the gold-standard scalpel to the latest lasers. Each modality has certain properties of its own. These properties may be suitable for certain dermatologic surgeries but not all, considering the depth of lesion and requirement of cosmesis.

Salient features and advantages and disadvantages of all the surgical modalities are listed next. This will facilitate the reader to better understand radiofrequency surgery.

Scalpel surgery
- Conventional method.
- Simplest of all modalities.
- Easy to arrange anywhere.
- Does not depend on electricity.
- Functions can be modified by changing the blades.
- Requires skill to operate.
- Intraoperative bleeding is a major disadvantage.
- Cannot be used effectively for superficial epidermal skin lesions.
- Very suitable for skin biopsy, incisional or excisional.
- Cut is thicker than radiofrequency and lasers.
- More postoperative pain and downtime compared to radiofrequency and lasers.
- Chances of scarring are more compared to radiofrequency and lasers.
- Suturing is a must for most cases.

Hyfrecator
- Small inexpensive equipment working on electricity.
- High frequency, high voltage but low current is used.
- Unipolar equipment (no antenna plate) is commonly used in dermatologic surgery.
- Portable, easy to shift, or carry to distant places for treatment.
- Functions of electrodesiccation, fulguration, and electrocoagulation are used.
- Good for superficial skin lesions of warts, skin tags, xanthelasma, and keratosis.
- Good for vascular skin lesions.
- Quick and effective modality for superficial skin lesions.
- Local anesthesia infiltration is not required in most lesions; only surface anesthesia suffices commonly.
- Skin lesions are literally destroyed by heat generation, which causes dehydration and necrosis, and the lesion remains sterile and stuck on, then desquamate in a week's time with negligible scarring.
- Vascular lesions may be treated repeatedly until final result.
- Postoperative pain is minimal with one-week downtime.
- Good cosmetic results.
- Not useful for skin biopsy as the lesion is destroyed, hence biopsy must be done prior to treatment.

Electrocautery
- Small, inexpensive equipment working on electricity.

- Portable, easy to carry anywhere.
- Popular among dermatologists.
- Low voltage, high current is used.
- Rheostat or resistor heats the electrode red-hot.
- Heat of electrocautery either excises or destroys the skin lesions.
- Good for coagulation, hence intraoperative bleeding is rare.
- Effective for vascular lesions.
- Good for superficial skin lesions like skin tags, xanthelasma, molluscum contagiosum, warts, granuloma pyogenicum, vascular lesions like hematoma, and hemostasis after excision of any skin lesion.
- Easy to operate.
- Some postoperative pain.
- Postoperative downtime is more.
- Postoperative healing is slow.
- Residual scarring is more likely to occur due to tissue destruction by red-hot electrode.
- Biopsy must be taken prior to electrocautery treatment.

Cryosurgery
- One of the simplest and popular methods.
- No electricity.
- Liquid nitrogen is used commonly.
- Containers and flasks containing liquid nitrogen need very careful handling.
- Local anesthesia is uncommonly required.
- Good results for superficial lesions of warts (cutaneous and mucosal), keratosis, skin tags, and molluscum contagiosum.
- Good results for basal cell carcinoma, superficial squamous cell carcinoma, and hemangiomas in experienced hands.
- Repeat treatments are necessary at intervals of 2 to 4 weeks for final results.
- Recurrence in warts and molluscum contagiosum possible.
- Can damage deeper tissues and superficial nerves in inexperienced hands.
- Posttreatment pain can be significant in some cases.
- Posttreatment hypopigmentation is common; takes a few weeks to months to recover.
- Posttreatment scarring is possible due to unpredictable level of freezing around treated lesions.

- Biopsy of treated lesion is possible by picking up the lesion with a punch or curette immediately after treatment, as the histology is not damaged in frozen lesion.

Radiofrequency surgery
- Among the latest effective methods for dermatologic surgery.
- Small portable equipment works on electricity.
- Good quality equipment is at least five times the cost of electrocautery.
- Equipment generates high-frequency radio waves above 1 MHz.
- The higher the radiofrequency, the finer the cut.
- Electrode remains cold throughout surgery, hence tissue damage is minimal.
- Pressureless precise incision is hallmark.
- Blending of cut and coagulation makes surgery dry and bloodless.
- Very fine cutting ability leads to very clean postoperative wounds, faster healing.
- Postoperative pain is much less.
- Postoperative scarring is negligible, virtually scarless removal of lesions.
- Very good for all kinds of dermatologic surgery.
- Requires operative skills.
- Very good alternative method for doing biopsy, as the lateral tissue thermal damage is minimal.

Ablative lasers
- Latest equipment for dermatologic surgery.
- Much larger in size, far more expensive (more than 20 times the cost of a good electrocautery).
- Works on electricity.
- Requires special training.
- Two major varieties, namely, Er:YAG and CO_2 lasers, are used.
- Cut is thicker than radiofrequency.
- Chances of charring are more in inexperienced hands.
- Dermatologic surgery with lasers requires good practice to avoid scarring.
- Postlaser pain is less compared to electrocautery and cryosurgery.
- Postlaser downtime similar to radiofrequency surgery.
- Er:YAG laser is good for superficial lesions only.

- CO_2 laser is good for superficial and deep skin lesions.
- CO_2 laser is good for vascular lesions, but not Er:YAG laser.
- Postinflammatory hyperpigmentation is more common after CO_2 laser than Er:YAG laser.
- Postlaser scarring is minimal.
- Laser teaching curve and experience is very important, without which chances of inferior results and cosmesis are very likely.
- Higher maintenance costs.
- Biopsy must be taken beforehand.

Some other dermatologic surgical modalities like the age-old chemical cautery and newer electrosurgery are not covered here. Chemical cautery is almost outdated and hardly practiced by today's doctors, except by practitioners in non-urban areas and classical clinical dermatologists. Electrosurgery equipment has features similar to radiofrequency surgery. Electrosurgical equipment has frequency less than 1 MHz and the results are inferior, though the equipment prices are much cheaper than radiofrequency surgery equipment. I consider radiofrequency surgery as nothing but "modern electrosurgery."

5

Why radiofrequency?

Dermatologic surgery has become more common in various clinics and hospitals because of the many factors discussed in previous chapters. Many small and large hospitals are taking interest in having this surgical service on their premises. They are ready to invest in equipment required to deliver the best results. There is an ever-increasing awareness among the general population regarding their skin lesions. Many seek advice for removal of their skin lesions either as treatment or to improve their appearance (for cosmetic purposes). Consultation for removal of unsightly skin lesions on the face or elsewhere has become extremely common.

In dermatologic surgery practice, most of the patients are not ill or unhealthy. These patients approach doctors for either one or more of the following needs:

- The lesions are very unsightly and spoiling their looks. These lesions include moles, keratosis, milia, ear keloids, keratoacanthoma, xanthelasma, syringoma, sebaceous cysts, and pyogenic granuloma.
- There is some kind of skin infection (e.g., verruca vulgaris, molluscum contagiosum, and condyloma acuminatum).
- The lesions are painful or cause discomfort in mobility, such as an infected skin tag or papilloma, corn, or callus.
- The lesions spoil facial appearance due to dotted hyperpigmented spots, as in freckles.
- Acne scars or deep crateriform scars.
- After hearing from some friends or knowing from media that such things can be easily done these days.
- Wish to look good by removing unsightly looking dermatosis papulosa nigra, senile comedones, syringoma, or capillary hemangioma.

- Senior citizens wishing to get rid of their skin tags or senile comedones on demand of their grandchildren or because they can afford to now.
- Wishing to spend on removing skin lesions on face in spite of nonaffordability only for cosmetic purpose.
- Referred to dermatologic surgery department from other doctors for removing skin lesions instead of to department of surgery.
- Need to do skin biopsy.

All the aforementioned indications, barring a few, were very commonly treated by general surgeons or otorhinolaryngologists or ophthalmologists when dermatologic surgery was not a specialty of its own. Today, due to a high following and superior techniques of dermatologic surgery, there is reverse flow, which has led the aforementioned specialties to learn from dermatologists.

The previous chapter dealt with all the available modalities for dermatologic surgery. When one considers the features marking the advantages and disadvantages of each modality, only one modality outsmarts all others, namely, radiofrequency surgery. It is hoped that the features of Table 5.1 will convince the reader of the advantages of radiofrequency surgery.

Let's review some of the technical criteria of radiofrequency surgery, which will give in-depth reasons to any practitioner for selecting this technique over others (Table 5.2).

Radiofrequency surgery holds a promise to be a superlative surgical tool for anyone who wishes to seriously take up dermatologic surgery. The points in both tables show that this modality is a marvelous refinement meant to deliver incomparable surgical applications with much better results.

Table 5.1 Advantages of radiofrequency surgery over other modalities

- Fulfillment of all criteria for office dermatologic surgery
- Small space occupancy of equipment
- Portability of equipment, hence can carry to hospitals if required
- Versatility of applications
- Price of equipment within reach of any new practitioner
- Very low maintenance costs
- Reusable electrodes, hence very low recurring costs
- Disposable electrodes also available
- Low power consumption
- Works easily on inverters in case of electricity failure
- Very good workmanship with good quality radiofrequency equipment
- Very good durability, can give service for years
- Can treat thousands of patients over many years

Table 5.2 Technical criteria of radiofrequency surgery

- Fine cutting ability, one of the finest cuts observed at about 3.8 to 4 MHz radiofrequency (Figures 5.1 and 5.2).[1]
- Cut and coagulation or blend facility to have bloodless operative field.
- Desiccation and fulguration modes for fine superficial work on skin.
- Good coagulation ability especially for vascular lesions or to arrest intraoperative bleeding.
- Sturdy tungsten metal electrodes with very thin dimensions.
- Large variety of electrodes, which gives practitioners multiplicity of applications.
- Easily bendable electrodes to reach certain lesions in orifices such as the nostrils, ear canal, oral cavity, and genitals.
- Insulated electrodes to prevent lateral tissue damage when working in orifices.
- Very clean postoperative wounds.
- Minimal postoperative pain.
- Faster postoperative healing.
- Sutureless surgery is very much possible.
- Virtually scarless surgery or with minimal scarring.

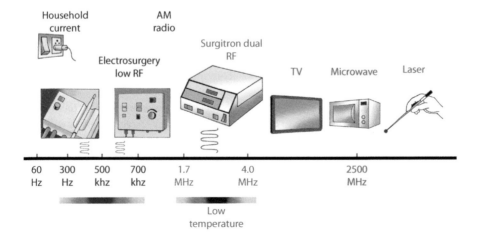

Figure 5.1 Placing 4 MHz radiofrequency unit on the graph of AC current frequencies in routine use.

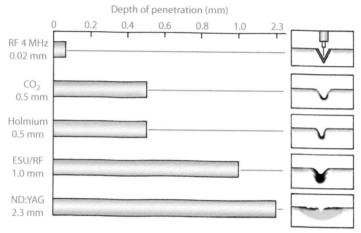

Figure 5.2 Comparison of tissue damage of 4 MHz radiofrequency surgery unit with various lasers in routine surgical practice.

Radiofrequency surgery is called a "virtual laser" by some because of so many properties matching with ablative lasers. But, I consider it a better alternative to ablative lasers because of its indisputable advantages over lasers. The most appealing benefits that make radiofrequency surgery a natural choice are the very fine cuts, almost bloodless operative field, negligible charring, very clean postoperative wounds, self-sterilizing, negligible lateral tissue thermal damage, virtually sutureless and scarless procedure, and affordable compared to lasers.

The following are some of the results of a survey given to dermatologists in India:

- More than 60% of dermatologists used the American-manufactured Ellman Surgitron, 5% used Korean or German or Bulgarian equipment, and all the rest had Indian-manufactured equipment from Dermaindia.
- Most of the applications covered in Chapters 13 and 14 were routinely done by these dermatologists, except those for lipoma excision, ingrown toenails, rhinophyma, capillary hemangioma, and skin biopsy.
- All agree that radiofrequency surgery has a unique place in dermatologic surgery, has low maintenance, has high patient satisfaction, and the least side effects.
- More than 50% do not use disposable electrodes; they sterilize electrodes before use.
- All dermatologists are happy with their results and would like to continue radiofrequency surgery in practice.
- Only three dermatologists have delegated radiofrequency surgery to their juniors or new dermatologists.

REFERENCE

1. Turner RJ, Cohen RA, Voet RL et al. Analysis of margins of cone biopsy specimens obtained with "cold knife," CO2 and Nd:YAG lasers and radiofrequency surgical unit. *J Reproductive Med* 1992; 607–610.

6

Practical tips for switching over to radiofrequency surgery

The previous chapter highlighted the practical points that have helped radiofrequency surgery to score over contemporary as well as the latest surgical techniques. Surgeons from any discipline of medicine always aim at delivering the best results. Their training institutes and the teaching faculty influence their practice. Overall, the techniques of scalpel, electrocautery, and cryosurgery have become commonplace in the majority of old and even many newer educational institutions. The use of newer techniques may get obstructed due to many unavoidable factors like educational curriculum changes, lack of budgeting, lack of teaching faculty, red-tapeism, and resistance to change. Let's discuss this in brief:

- *Educational curriculum changes*—These are the most difficult to overcome, because the decisions for this are made at the governmental level where the influence of medical faculty is lacking. Also, dermatology is a specialty that has gained importance only over the past decade, at least in India. The situation is likely to be far better in Western countries where curriculum updating takes place at a faster pace.
- *Lack of budgeting*—The allotment and sanctioning of budgets is a matter of governmental authorities where again medical faculty lacks influence. Additionally, here again dermatology has only started gaining in the past decade. Private institutions are way ahead in investing.
- *Lack of teaching faculty*—Teaching faculty need regular updating at all educational institutions, which is not happening in developing

countries. Also, unless institutions invest in newer gadgets, how can teachers be updated?
- *Red-tapeism*—Occasionally, this can become a much greater obstruction to sanctioning of the budgets to update the surgical departments.
- *Resistance to change*—Any major change is always resisted by the old medical faculty. The reasons for this include hurting of egos to apprehension of learning and implementing newer techniques.

In this chapter, I have made an effort to help practitioners make a smooth transition to radiofrequency surgery. A clinician having a surgical practice of at least 5 years (but not using radiofrequency method) should not find it difficult to switch to dermatologic surgery with radiofrequency. Following are some very simple and easy-to-learn tips to facilitate this transition.

FROM SCALPEL TO RADIOFREQUENCY (RF) SURGERY

When we consider the close comparison between the two modalities of Table 6.1, practitioners who are only used to scalpel surgery can very quickly gain expertise in radiofrequency surgery by following these tips and tricks:

- Learn to use radiofrequency surgery technique on meat pieces for practice first.
- Get thoroughly acquainted with mode and power settings as well as selection of electrode (refer to Chapter 8).

Table 6.1 Switch from scalpel to RF surgery

Scalpel surgery	RF surgery
Cutting tissue requires pressure	Pressureless cutting of tissue
Bleeding follows any cut	Bleeding well controlled during cut
Tissue cutting is not fine	Tissue cutting is fine
Lesion is usually excised in toto	Lesion is usually excised piece by piece
Excising vascular lesions requires electrocoagulation	Excising vascular lesions is facilitated due to blend mode and separate electrocoagulation mode as well as bipolar coagulation if required
Suturing is commonly required after excision	Suturing is not required commonly after excision
Shaping or sculpting of tissues not possible	Shaping or sculpting of tissues is possible on low power
Very difficult to finely excise superficial lesions	Very good for fine superficial excisions
Cut precision is difficult	Cut precision is absolutely sure
Time required may be more due to bleeding and suturing	Time required is less due to bloodless operative field

- Hold the electrode and only slide through the desired tissue to cut without pressure like a hot knife through butter once you have selected the mode.
- The inability to cut means the power setting is low. Pressure should never be applied if there is inability to cut.
- Pressure applied will create damage and cause very deep cuts, complicating the matter.
- Thin multiple cuts should be attempted instead of in toto removal.
- A bloodless operative field allows the practitioner to judge the correct depth of the removed lesion.
- Use the blend mode for vascular lesions.
- Pressure hemostasis can suffice many a times.
- The technique to treat superficial epidermal lesions has to be learned separately (refer to Chapter 8).
- Incision and excision biopsy is possible.

FROM ELECTROCAUTERY TO RF SURGERY

The comparison of Table 6.2 shows that any practitioner who is conversant and familiar with electrocautery will benefit more using radiofrequency surgery. This switchover is not difficult. Most important, the treating electrode of electrocautery is always hot, whereas the electrode of radiofrequency surgery is always cold, hence with

practice of making paintbrush-like strokes (refer to Chapter 8), any practitioner can deliver much better results. The tips to use radiofrequency surgery best are given next:

- Use the correct electrode, mode, and optimum power to excise lesions.
- Use multiple strokes and remove lesions piece by piece instead of destruction as in electrocautery.
- The blend mode helps control intraoperative bleeding and is best for vascular skin lesions.
- Superficial skin lesions should be treated very finely at minimum power to just dehydrate lesions.
- Incision or excision biopsy is well performed in one stroke at optimum power.

The reader should refer Chapter 8 for all the aforementioned points before using radiofrequency surgery instead of electrocautery. The advantages of using radiofrequency surgery outweighs the benefits of electrocautery in all respects because not only do the applications increase but even the results are superior.

FROM CRYOSURGERY TO RF SURGERY

A practitioner expert in cryosurgery can easily switch over to radiofrequency surgery for the betterment of practice as well as expanding the

Table 6.2 Switch from electrocautery to RF surgery

Electrocautery	RF surgery
Hot electrode cuts lesion	Cold electrode cuts lesion by generating heat at electrode tip
Hot electrode destroys lesion	Cold electrode does not destroy lesion, cuts only at electrode tip
Cut is never fine	Cut is always fine
Procedure is always bloodless due to hot electrode	Procedure is usually bloodless
Postoperative wound is not very clean, may be charred	Postoperative wound is very clean, there is no charring
Vascular lesions easily tackled	Vascular lesions can be very well tackled
Postoperative pain is more	Postoperative pain is much less
Postoperative healing is slow	Postoperative healing is faster
Postoperative scarring very common	Postoperative scarring is negligible
Superficial lesions can be tackled well	Superficial lesions treated the best
Skin biopsy not possible	Skin biopsy is very much possible

Table 6.3 Switch from cryosurgery to RF surgery

Cryosurgery	RF surgery
Works on principle of destruction of tissues (tissue necrosis) with extremely cold (subzero) temperature	Works on principle of thermal necrosis of tissues using radiofrequency waves
Difficult to control depth of destruction, requires good experience	Can control level and depth of tissue removal precisely
Can damage lateral tissues as well as melanocytes leading to hypopigmentation	Unlikely to damage lateral tissues or melanocytes, but postoperative hyperpigmentation is common on brown or dark skin
Skin biopsy is possible, as freezing preserves tissue architecture	Skin biopsy is easily done without major tissue damage

applications (Table 6.3). The following tips will guide practitioners to facilitate this transition:

- After getting acquainted with the radiofrequency surgery technique, practitioners must be aware that they are using high temperature to destroy or cut lesions and this high temperature can cause burns if not careful.
- Holding of electrodes and their proper use can give very satisfactory results.
- Superficial skin lesions whiten (dehydrate) with fine touch of electrode tip.
- Use cut or blend mode for excising lesions.
- Skin biopsy can be performed very easily.

Radiofrequency surgery can replace cryosurgery because of its many benefits that allow treatment of all common superficial and deep skin lesions with wonderful cosmesis.

FROM ABLATIVE LASERS TO RF SURGERY

Switching from ablative lasers to radiofrequency surgery is not difficult (see Table 6.4). Here the practitioner who is an expert in using ablative lasers must bear in mind that he or she is conversant with a technology that is operated from a certain distance and the scab needs to be removed after every pass to

Table 6.4 Switch from ablative lasers to RF surgery

Ablative lasers	RF surgery
Photothermal destruction of tissues	Electrothermal destruction of tissues
Tissue cutting is fine	Tissue cutting can be finer than lasers
Depth control requires good experience	Depth control easily achieved due to tactile advantage
Tissue charring may occur	Tissue charring is almost nil
Skin biopsy is impossible	Skin biopsy is an advantage

get proper judgment of the depth of lesion removed. Whereas in radiofrequency surgery, this depth is very easily ascertained as the electrode removes the tissues layer by layer very finely without charring.

Here are the tips for switching over:

- Always remove lesions layer by layer with radiofrequency surgery at minimum required or optimum power.

- Use blend mode if necessary.
- There are no preset parameters; these differ with type of lesion.
- Undercorrection is the aim to prevent complications.
- Skin biopsy is an advantage.

7

Fundamental features
of radiofrequency surgery

The clinical effects of radiofrequency (RF) surgery are very much dependent upon the physical characteristics of the equipment as developed by the manufacturer. Among the physical characteristics, the clinical tissue effects depend upon the combination of RF parameters and the method of application to the tissues.

PHYSICAL CHARACTERISTICS[1]

Radiofrequency in physics relates to the radio waves in the electromagnetic spectrum from 3 kHz to 300 GHz. But, in medicine only those between 200 kHz and 40 MHz are used. At radiofrequency below 100 kHz the nerve and muscle stimulation is very high, which can cause major or fatal side effects. The dermatological effects are observed best at frequencies above 500 kHz.

The principle of radiofrequency surgery is that the human tissues are heated to the extent of necrosis leading to a cut due to tissue impedance to radio waves delivered through the electrode. While the tissues are exposed to an alternating current (AC) at frequencies higher than 500 kHz there are chances of tissue burns or charring. To minimize the lateral tissue damage and to minimize chances of charring while doing surgery, there are some important physical parameters that when understood one can deliver the best results.

The physical parameters of utmost importance when using radiofrequency surgery are the following:

- *Frequency of radio waves*—The higher the frequency above 1 MHz, the finer the cut, that is, the lateral heat dispersion is inversely proportional to the radiofrequency.
- *Electrode size*—The larger the size of the electrode, the more the lateral heat dispersion, that is, the lateral heat dispersion is directly proportional to the size of electrodes.
- *Time of tissue contact*—The higher the electrode contact time of the treated tissue, the more the lateral tissue damage, that is, lateral heat dispersion is directly proportional to time of electrode–tissue contact.
- *Radiofrequency power*—Optimum power gives the best results, that is, lateral tissue damage is directly proportional to power.
- *Waveform*—A fully filtered or cut waveform is least damaging to lateral tissues, whereas the blend (cut + coag) and electrocoagulation waveforms are more damaging to lateral tissues.

The practical applications of the physical characteristics can be summed up as follows: The radiofrequency of the equipment used will always remain constant in all procedures. Hence, to deliver the best results, one has to control the other parameters mentioned earlier. The higher the lateral tissue thermal dispersion, the higher the tissue damage. To deliver the best results, select the smallest or the thinnest electrode, use the cut or blend mode, keep the contact time of the electrode with tissue to a minimum, and use minimum required power.

BIOLOGICAL CHARACTERISTICS

Advancements in the knowledge of electromagnetism and electronics have helped in development of newer RF equipment having different functions to suit and expand applications in clinical practice. This has been possible by developing these functions to suit the practitioner's needs when operating on skin.

When operating on skin any dermatologic surgeon expects the following:

- Cutting should be fine.
- Bloodless cutting is preferable.
- Coagulation ability after excision and for removing vascular lesions.
- Ability to work very finely on superficial skin lesions.
- Avoid postoperative sequelae of scarring.

The aforementioned expectations of a dermatologic surgeon are fulfilled successfully by the generation of *waveforms*. Refer to the upcoming section on functionality for the details about waveforms and their exact usefulness for versatility of applications. In brief, each waveform causes a different biologic outcome ranging from dehydration (electrodesiccation) to destruction or hemostasis (electrocoagulation) to tissue cutting (electrosection).

All radiofrequency surgery units are *monopolar*. Monopolar RF devices have an active electrode used for treating and a return electrode or ground plate/antenna plate that completes the

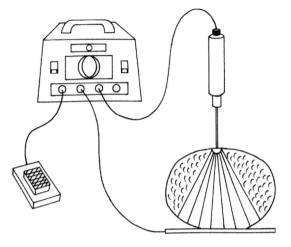

Figure 7.1 Electrical circuit including patient (how electrical current flows during surgery). (Modified from Brown J, *Minor Surgery: A Text and Atlas*, 4th edition, Arnold Publishers, 2000, p. 312, Figure 42.1.)

electrical circuit. The treated patient is part of the electrical circuit. These units are also described as *monopolar and biterminal* (Figure 7.1). These functions are used for excision, destruction, and coagulation.

The same radiofrequency surgery unit can be used without connecting the antenna plate. This application is termed *monopolar monoterminal*. Here, the radio waves generated are delivered through the active electrode at the lesion. This function is used only for superficial epidermal lesions at optimum power. This dehydrates and destroys the lesion, which can be immediately peeled off or allowed to peel off later. This is further described later as electrodesiccation and electrofulguration.

The principle on which the radiofrequency surgery works is the *electrothermal effect*. The high-frequency radio waves are generated by the AC current when they contact the skin. The electrode tip is always cold. The electrode tip upon reaching the skin delivers the radio waves, which travel through the human body toward the antenna plate. The skin and subcutaneous tissues resist the passage of radio waves. The resistance or impedance to the passage of radio waves creates subcellular water molecular friction. Water molecular friction generates tremendous heat to make subcellular water boil (see Figures 7.2 to 7.5). The generated heat dehydrates all concerned cells leading to necrosis and splitting of epidermis, dermis, and subcutaneous tissues as the case may be. The generated heat also coagulates proteins, coagulates blood vessels, and cuts nerve endings. The injury created by radio waves will depend on the waveform used, electrode tip size (spot size), and power used. In waveforms of electrodesiccation and electrofulguration, the absence of an antenna plate makes radio waves concentrate only over surface lesions without traversing through the body.

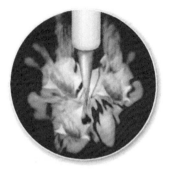

Figure 7.4 Consequent heat generation causes tissue necrosis.

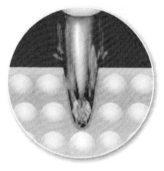

Figure 7.5 Electrode cuts through causing very thin splitting of tissues (fine cut).

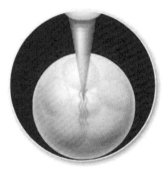

Figure 7.2 Electrode touches skin.

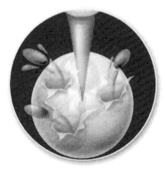

Figure 7.3 Tissue resistance leads to boiling of intracellular and extracellular water molecules.

The main advantages of monopolar RF devices are

- The thermal effects are predictable at the active electrode tip.
- The thermal effect is possible because of the ability to concentrate thermal energy on a small portion of the tissue to be treated and abrupt reduction of the same energy away from the electrode tip through the tissue toward the antenna plate. This limits the heat damage away from the electrode tip.

Figure 7.6 gives a clear idea of these advantages.

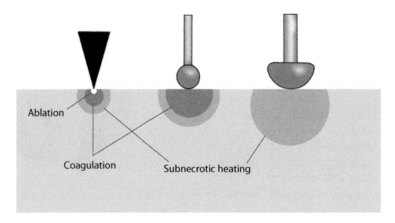

Figure 7.6 RF spot-size effects on tissues. (Modified from Duncan DI, Kreindel M, Basic radiofrequency: Physics and safety and applications to aesthetic medicine, in *Radiofrequency in Cosmetic Dermatology*, edited by M Lapidoth, S Halachmi. Basel: Karger; 2015, p. 8, Figure 6.)

EQUIPMENT DETAILS[2]

Any radiofrequency surgery equipment consists of the following (also see Figure 7.7):

- Radiofrequency generator or unit
- Handpiece (with or without activating switch)
- Antenna plate or ground plate (nonmetal)
- Foot pedal to activate unit
- Electrodes of various shapes and sizes (Figure 7.8)

FUNCTIONALITY

Any dermatologic surgeon who uses radiofrequency equipment ought to be well acquainted with the functional features of the radiofrequency. These are tabulated in detail in Table 7.1.[3]

The four common applications[4] are shown in Figures 7.9 to 7.12 for easy understanding.

The key to optimal use of radiofrequency in dermatologic surgery practice is for the practitioner to understand the predictable biologic effects

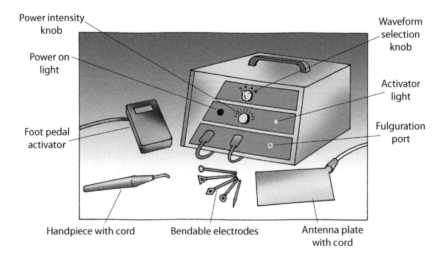

Figure 7.7 Radiofrequency surgery equipment details.

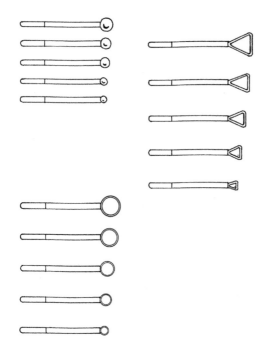

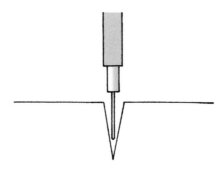

Figure 7.9 Electrosection, a very fine cut, cuts exactly where electrode touches.

Figure 7.8 Different electrodes in various sizes.

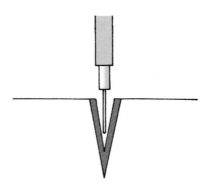

Figure 7.10 Blend (Cut + Cog: 50%–50%) gives bloodless operative field.

Table 7.1 Basic waveforms, lateral heat spread, uses

Waveform	Electrode function	Lateral heat spread	Applications
Fully filtered, fully rectified "pure cut"	Electrosection: 90% cut, 10% coag	Least	Incisions, excisions, biopsy
Fully rectified	Blend: 50% cut, 50% coag	Medium	Incisions, excisions where bleeding is expected
Partially rectified	Electrocoagulation: 90% coag, 10% cut	Most	Hemostasis, epilation, telangiectasia
Marked damped spark gap	Electrodessication, fulguration	Medium	Superficial epidermal lesions

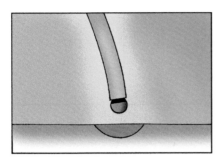

Figure 7.11 Electrocoagulation, for hemostasis.

and select the appropriate waveform for best clinical outcome in the particular clinical situation encountered.

Let me explain this with some examples:

- Superficial epidermal lesions on the face are best tackled with electrodessication at low power.
- Verruca plana on face are best tackled with electrodessication at low power.
- Vascular lesions anywhere are best tackled with the blend mode at optimum power.
- Hyperkeratotic lesions, such as corns and calluses, are best tackled with electrosection because it cuts the best, followed by the blend mode to clear debris and give a clean postoperative wound. Electrocoagulation is applied if required.
- Electrosection is used most commonly for excision as well as biopsy.
- Electrocoagulation is not used alone generally.

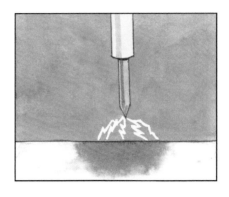

Figure 7.12 Fulguration, RF waves jump a small distance for superficial destruction of lesion.

REFERENCES

1. Pollack SV. How electrosurgical devices work. In: *Electrosurgery of the Skin*, 1st edition, New York, Churchill Livingston, 1991, 7–13.
2. Pfenninger JS, Fowler GC. Radiofrequency surgery (modern electrosurgery). In: *Procedures for Primary Care Physicians*, 2nd edition, 2003, 213–224.
3. Deshpande B. Radiofrequency treatment ablative and non-ablative. In: *Practical Manual of Cosmetic Dermatology and Surgery*, 1st edition, New Delhi, Mehta Publishers, 2010, 377–388.
4. Pollack SV. Electrodessication, electrofulguration, electroepilation. In: *Electrosurgery of the Skin*, 1st edition, New York, Churchill Livingston, 1991, 31–68.

8

Radiofrequency surgery operative skills: Tips and tricks to master the technique

The hallmarks of radiofrequency surgery are

- High radiofrequency
- Low electrode temperature

Both these features make this surgical modality safe. The higher the radiofrequency, the better and finer the cut.[1] The higher radiofrequency also is safer from the fact that it does not cause nerve and muscle stimulation, which occurs with lower radiofrequency waves. Low temperature means "cold electrode," thus minimizing the chances of tissue destruction and making the technique safe.

The method of using radiofrequency surgery remains the same whether it is used in dermatologic surgery, dentistry, general surgery, ophthalmology, gynecology, proctology, neurosurgery, or spine surgery. Chapter 6 provided tips for switching over for different faculty surgeons as well as orthodox and newer dermatologists.

The learning curve for radiofrequency surgery involves a few tips and tricks that are connected with the full knowledge of the fundamental features covered in Chapter 7. In dermatologic surgery, the primary concern is the skin surface, which has aesthetic value whether it is over exposed area or covered area. Patients today are always concerned about postoperative scarring.

The tips and tricks given in the following are for the general use of radiofrequency dermatologic surgery. Yet, when put into practice any

practitioner can be best assured of superior results. In addition, more gems for achieving aesthetically superior results are given in Chapter 15.

Tips and tricks to master radiofrequency surgery techniques are listed in Table 8.1 and briefly explained next:

- *Pressureless incision*—Figure 8.1 provides a very good idea about how such an incision will cut the skin and subcutaneous tissues, resulting in a very clean cut as though the tissues have just split off without charring or unevenness.
- *Fine and light strokes (feather touch or paintbrush like)*—Figure 8.2 will give a very good idea about how to use feather-touch strokes to delicately excise the skin lesions for delivering the best aesthetic result. These strokes are made until the whole lesion is fully removed; judgment of the depth of skin lesions is well understood while making the fine strokes. Once the excision is over, the blending is also done with fine strokes. I would like to define this as "portrait-shading strokes" (Figure 8.3).
- *Appropriate electrode size and shape*—Figure 8.4 gives an idea of different electrodes with their shapes and sizes. The thinner the electrode, the finer the cut. The appropriate shape to match the skin lesion is also important for best results.
- *Appropriate waveform selection*—Chapter 7 discussed the available waveforms and their

Table 8.1 Tips to master radiofrequency surgery

- Pressureless incision
- Fine and light strokes (feather touch or paintbrush like)
- Appropriate electrode size
- Appropriate waveform selection
- Appropriate power setting
- Antenna plate position
- Hydration of skin lesion
- Interval between two strokes

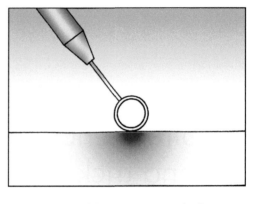

Figure 8.3 Very delicate "portrait-shading strokes" where the electrode barely touches skin (masterstroke of radiofrequency surgery).

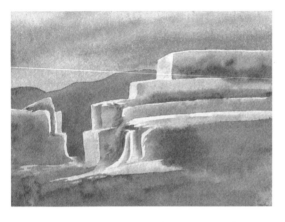

Figure 8.1 Picture simulates how pressureless incision cuts tissues as though it splits.

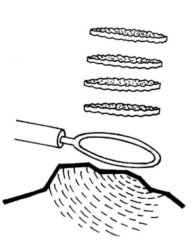

Figure 8.2 Shave excision.

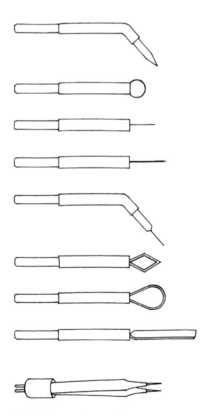

Figure 8.4 Various electrodes.

applications. Waveform selection is of paramount importance for flawless dermatologic surgery.

- *Appropriate power setting*—There are no fixed power settings for particular skin lesions, though some settings can be fixed for indications of desiccation and fulguration. For various skin lesions tackled by excision, only a range of power settings can be given as guidelines. These settings will vary for different skin lesions as well as the equipment used. Optimum power always gives the best operability and thus best results. Optimum power settings for practitioners are individualized and come by experience.

- *Antenna plate position*—The antenna plate is nonmetal and is not required to touch the patient's skin. It should be kept close to the site of operation for best results.

- *Hydration of skin lesion*—Radiofrequency surgery works on principle of vaporization and hence while cutting, the skin lesion should be well hydrated so that it is moist enough for the electrode tip to literally glide through without efforts or dragging of tissues. Dry lesions will resist cutting. Hydration is not required ideally for superficial lesions tackled using desiccation and fulguration.

- *Interval between two strokes*—It is advisable to avoid hurried strokes while excising to avoid tissue charring. There is no rule about how much interval, but strokes given one after another should be at comfortable intervals that will not allow tissue charring.

I have conducted more than 50 comprehensive radiofrequency surgery training workshops in India at many local, regional, and national conferences, as well as in Noble Hospital, Pune, India (Figures 8.5 to 8.7). Practitioners from different surgical faculties like general surgery, otorhinolaryngology, ophthalmology, and plastic surgery in addition to dermatology have attended

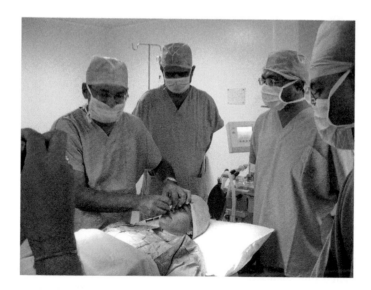

Figure 8.5 Briefing before starting workshop.

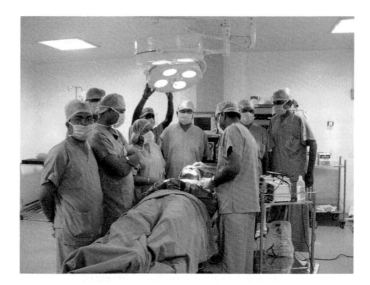

Figure 8.6 Introducing technique before workshop.

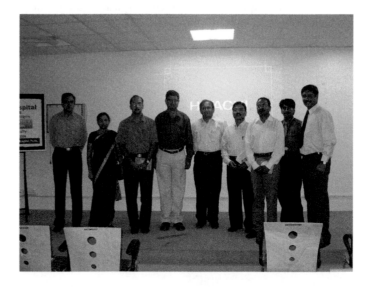

Figure 8.7 Hands-on training workshop for 5 to 10 practitioners at a time.

my workshops, which had certificate courses as well. I also conducted one such workshop in Cairo, Egypt, for my Arab medical colleagues. These workshops covered surgical and nonsurgical (skin tightening) applications of 4 MHz radiofrequency.

REFERENCE

1. Maness WL, Roeber FW, Clarke RE et al. Histological evaluation of electrosurgery with varying frequency and waveforms. *J Prosthetic Dent* 1978; 40:304–308.

9

Precautions and safety measures

Radiofrequency surgery equipment is an electrical gadget. Hence, the precautions and safety measures related with the hazards of electric current are the main concern. The manufacturer always takes full safety measures not to allow any leakage of electric current during the use of the equipment. Yet, there are certain issues one should know before giving the treatment.

PATIENT SAFETY ISSUES

Cardiac pacemakers and radiofrequency surgery

Cardiac pacemakers have an electric circuit (battery operated). Today's pacemakers are far better protected from electrical cross circuits than a few decades back, yet it is always safe to avoid radiofrequency surgery in such patients. The radio waves travel through the body of the patient toward the antenna plate as mentioned on page 24, Figure 7.1, Chapter 7. These waves have the potential to affect the pacemaker function. Some practitioners advise either to keep the antenna plate far away from the vicinity of the pacemaker to avoid the radio waves disturbing the pacemaker circuit or delivering radiofrequency waves in bursts of less than 5 seconds to avoid the same problem. *A prior consent from the patient's cardiologist is a must before performing radiofrequency surgery for such patients.* I prefer avoiding radiofrequency surgery in such patients. If needed, these patients can be safely treated with other modalities. I have included a statement in my informed consent forms that confirms the patient does not have a cardiac pacemaker. This form has to be duly signed separately for our safety.[1-3] Refer to Chapter 11 for more information about the consent form.

Electrical shock

It is advisable to check that the patient's skin does not have a direct contact with any metal, which makes the patient prone to electrical shock. Ideally, a dental metal implant or some other metal objects like watches, jewelry, earrings, and spectacles have not led to electrical shock so far in my practice. It is impractical to ask patients to remove everything before office dermatologic surgery. Dental metal implants are fixed. I have observed that the patient reports some heat or pain where there is close skin or mucosal contact of metal. This is more common if the surgical site is in the vicinity of the metal as the radio waves delivered from the active electrode while passing through the body toward the antenna plate heat the metal.

Fire or burns

Radiofrequency surgical procedures conducted in the presence of alcohol-based antiseptic can cause accidental burns to the patient. It is thus advisable to avoid them prior to such surgery. Since alcohol-based antiseptic is probably among the cheapest for preoperative sterilization, I prefer using them but allow sufficient time for the solution to evaporate and the area to fully dry (approximately 2 to 3 minutes). Oxygen also can cause fire, but this is only applicable to the operating theater setup. A patient's bowel gas (methane) is highly inflammable, hence proper care should be taken when working in perianal, perineal, and genital areas.

PRACTITIONER SAFETY ISSUES

Electrical shock

Practitioners need to be very careful when handling electrodes. The electrodes must always be fully and tightly inserted (screwed inside or press fitted as per the handpiece). The insulation of the electrode has to go inside the handpiece. In case of loose fitting or if the insulation has worn out, there is always a possibility of electrical shock to the practitioners. Wearing latex rubber gloves gives full protection from such accidents.

Microorganism transmission

Practitioners are exposed to intact viral particles while working on patients, especially those who have viral warts or molluscum contagiosum. Intact viral particles have been recovered from smoke plumes generated during electrosection and electrocoagulation. A smoke evacuator with its smoke absorbing head should be held close to the surgical site (approximately 2 to 5 cm) by an assistant during such operations where there is viral infection. Wearing of surgical masks in addition will serve to protect as well. Additionally, when working under a circular magnifying lens, the lens itself can act as a barrier for easy transmission of these particles from patients.[1–3]

REFERENCES

1. Sebben JE. Electrosurgery and cardiac pacemakers. *J Am Acad Dermatol* 1983; 9:457–463.
2. Pollack SV. Potential hazards of electrosurgery. In: *Electrosurgery of the Skin*, 1st edition, New York, Churchill Livingstone, 1991, 71–72.
3. Sebben JE. The hazards of electrosurgery. *J Am Acad Dermatol* 1987; 16:869–872.

10

Radiofrequency surgery rehearsal or practice sessions

I strongly recommend rehearsal or practice sessions on pieces of meat or chicken before starting your work on patients. The time allotted to practice will never go to waste, in fact, it will cut short the learning curve for the new user. In this chapter I have made an effort to practically demonstrate the use of all modes or waveforms of radiofrequency surgery equipment. This will thus make the switch from other surgical modalities (refer to Chapter 6) much easier. Additionally, practice on meat or chicken will give the feel of the technique as well as the visual impact of the treated tissues. This will facilitate the applications dramatically.

Radiofrequency surgery has become very familiar with medical practitioners. Hence, many medical equipment manufacturers have invested in developing their own radiofrequency equipment. There is a lot of good quality equipment on the market. Radiofrequency surgery devices have been manufactured in many countries including the United States, Germany, South Korea, India, China, and Taiwan. This equipment varies in their parameters like the exact radiofrequency delivered (1 to 4 MHz), power, and the quality of cut and coagulation waveforms. I have used the Ellman Surgitron from the United States, hence here I am specifying the parameters accordingly. There will be some variations in the power settings when using other radiofrequency equipment.

PRACTICE SESSION SUGGESTIONS AND TIPS

The following items will be required for a practice session[1]:

- Radiofrequency surgery equipment
- Electrodes such as a straight needle electrode, fine wire electrode (Vari-Tip), broad needle electrode, wire loop electrode, ball electrode, round blade or flat disclike Surgipen electrode
- Surgical gloves
- Tissue forceps
- Normal saline bottle for moistening tissue
- Four to five sufficiently large pieces of chicken or meat
- Small, fine-bristle paintbrush and dark watercolor (only for understanding)

Before a practice session ensure the following:

- Always confirm proper fitting of electrode in the handpiece. The insulated portion of the electrode must be fully inside the handpiece; there must be no gap left (Figures 10.1 and 10.2).
- Always start from a lower power to reach optimum while cutting.
- The angle at which the electrode is held, contact time of electrode to tissue, dragging

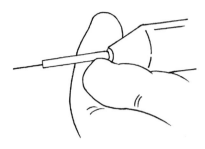

Figure 10.1 Electrode insulation must be inserted fully inside the headpiece. (Modified from Pollack SV, Laboratory exercises, in *Electrosurgery of the Skin*, 1st edition, New York, Churchill Livingstone, 1991, p. 75, Figure 14.1.)

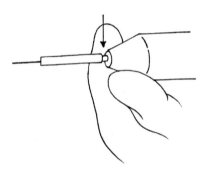

Figure 10.2 An incompletely inserted electrode can cause electric shock. (Modified from Pollack SV, Laboratory exercises, in *Electrosurgery of the Skin*, 1st edition, New York, Churchill Livingstone, 1991, p. 75, Figure 14.2.)

of electrode in tissue, and sparking at the time of cut are important points to be keenly observed.
- Always moisten the meat piece before working on it.
- As a matter of pictorial way of understanding, which can make a concrete impact on the learning practitioner, I recommend trying it yourself with the use of a fine-bristle paintbrush with India ink on a drawing paper in the way shown in Figure 10.3.

You also need to ensure the following when getting ready for a practice session:

- Radiofrequency surgery equipment is connected to the mains electricity supply.
- Antenna plate is connected into the socket marked for it.

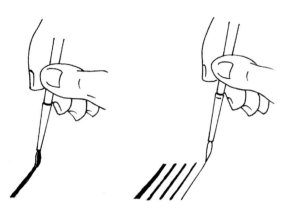

Figure 10.3 A fine bristle paintbrush is comparable to a fine electrode (for thinnest cut). (Modified from Pollack SV, Laboratory exercises, in *Electrosurgery of the Skin*, 1st edition, New York, Churchill Livingstone, 1991, p. 80, Figure 14.9.)

- Handpiece is connected into the socket marked for it.
- Foot pedal is connected and kept on the floor.
- Meat piece wrapped in cellophane is opened.
- Antenna plate is kept underneath the meat piece.
- Equipment is switched on.

APPLICATIONS OF WAVEFORMS

The next sections describe the exercises to be carried out for each of the waveforms used.

Electrosection or fully filtered current

This is a pure cutting current (waveform). Electrically, it is a continuous flow of nonpulsating high radiofrequency AC current. This is known to produce the least amount of lateral heat dispersion and hence the least tissue destruction. This is due to its properties of microsmooth dissection.

- After primary preparation, as given earlier, a straight needle electrode is selected and inserted fully inside the handpiece. Power is set to a minimum of 2. The electrode is held perpendicular to the meat piece and touched gently to cut. At this low power, generally the electrode does not cut at all or will cut with some effort, but the cut is shabby and tissue pieces will stick to the electrode. This is the effect of low power.

- Increase the power to 8 to 10 and make a cut. The resultant cut will be with sparking and some charring. This cut is not a good cut. It is inferior and more likely to cause tissue charring and damage leading to side effects or inferior cosmesis in practice. This power is very high.
- After exploring different powers from 2 to 10, you will be able to find the optimum power setting for cutting the meat piece. The optimum power will allow a microsmooth or fine cut without charring and sparking. This power could be between 3 and 5. This power will help with pressureless incision and effortless cutting. The cuts made with such power will look very clean and fine as though the tissue has just split. Tissue will never stick to electrode.
- Try the same using the fine wire or Vari-Tip electrode.
- Try also the round loop electrode. You can try cutting with the loop by holding the tissue with forceps. You can practice with the loop to make superficial and deeper excisions. The loop electrode is used very commonly in dermatologic surgery (Figures 10.4 to 10.6).

This waveform is best for all kinds of surgical incisions and excisions, from removing of corns, keratoses, papillomas, acrochordons, moles, and warts to doing a biopsy. Electrodes are changed according to the need. Hemostasis has to be done separately.

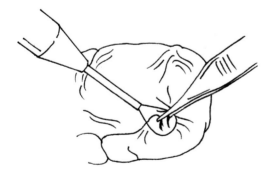

Figure 10.4 Holding a meat piece with forceps to cut with a round loop electrode. (Modified from Pollack SV, Laboratory exercises, in *Electrosurgery of the Skin*, 1st edition, New York, Churchill Livingstone, 1991, p. 80, Figure 14.10.)

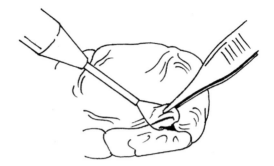

Figure 10.5 Cutting with optimum power. (Modified from Pollack SV, Laboratory exercises, in *Electrosurgery of the Skin*, 1st edition, New York, Churchill Livingstone, 1991, p. 81, Figure 14.11.)

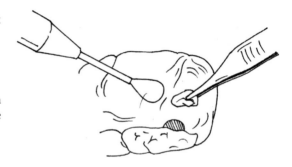

Figure 10.6 Optimum power cuts fast and smooth. (Modified from Pollack SV, Laboratory exercises, in *Electrosurgery of the Skin*, 1st edition, New York, Churchill Livingstone, 1991, p. 81, Figure 14.12.)

Blend current or fully rectified current

This is a blended cutting current (waveform). There is a minute pulsating effect incorporated. This helps simultaneous hemostasis. The efficiency of pure cutting waveform is thus blunted marginally. There is some lateral heat dispersion, which may cause mild charring. Due to the pulsating nature, the power required for cutting will have to be increased.

- After primary preparation as described earlier, a straight needle electrode is inserted fully into the handpiece. The power is set to 2. Cutting will hardly occur at this low power. Increasing the power to 4 may allow some cutting but is likely to cause dragging of the electrode in tissue. Increasing the power to 5 or 6 will allow increased RF fluence and allow easy and smooth cutting.

- A few differences noted while cutting with the blend current are that the power required for smooth cutting is more than the pure cut waveform; the pulsating nature of this current will be felt while cutting (tactile quality); the resultant cut will be slightly thicker compared to electrosection; and there could be mild superficial charring.
- Try using other electrodes for practice.

This waveform is best for all kinds of incisions and excisions where there are chances of intraoperative bleeding. This waveform will thus provide a bloodless operative field to the practitioner. This is helpful when removing vascular skin lesions. It is better to avoid this waveform on the face unless required due to a slightly inferior cosmetic outcome.

Electrocoagulation or partially rectified current

This waveform is a pulsating or interrupted AC current. The pulsations are very well perceived while operating. This thus blunts the cutting nature and disperses more lateral tissue heat. There is the possibility of more charring and tissue destruction. This waveform should never be used for cutting.

- After primary preparation as mentioned earlier, the smallest of the ball electrode is inserted fully into the handpiece. The power is kept at 3 to 4. The electrode is allowed to deeply press into the meat piece and remain touching it. Surprisingly, there will not be any reaction (Figure 10.7).
- Now, without increasing power, lift the electrode and lightly retouch the surface of the meat piece. You will immediately perceive a pulsating current. This is the feature of the partially rectified waveform. Simultaneously, you will observe the charring of the tissue where the electrode touched the meat piece (Figure 10.8).
- Increase power to above 6 to observe the effects of more RF fluence. There will be more lateral heat dispersion leading to more charring of the meat piece; consequently there will be more tissue destruction (Figure 10.9).

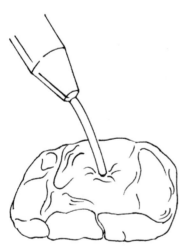

Figure 10.7 Electrocoagulation cannot be done by simply pushing the electrode continuously into meat. (Modified from Pollack SV, Laboratory exercises, in *Electrosurgery of the Skin*, 1st edition, New York, Churchill Livingstone, 1991, p. 76, Figure 14.3.)

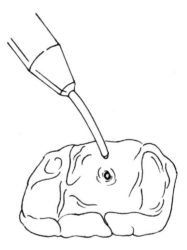

Figure 10.8 Electrocoagulation occurs best by lightly touching the meat piece. (Modified from Pollack SV, Laboratory exercises, in *Electrosurgery of the Skin*, 1st edition, New York, Churchill Livingstone, 1991, p. 76, Figure 14.4.)

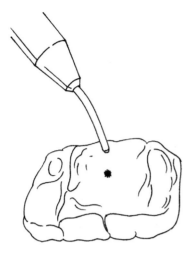

Figure 10.9 Electrocoagulation causes charring of tissue. (Modified from Pollack SV, Laboratory exercises, in *Electrosurgery of the Skin*, 1st edition, New York, Churchill Livingstone, 1991, p. 77, Figure 14.5.)

When using this waveform, always ensure that it is used for hemostasis of vascular tissue or arresting bleeding after excision. Always use it in the same manner as described. Use of this waveform for facial lesions should be avoided unless really required due to possibility of scarring. Besides hemostasis, this waveform is used for epilation and telangiectasia; please refer to further chapters for these applications.

Electrodessication and electrofulguration

This waveform is a modification of electrocoagulation where the antenna plate is not in circuit (monopolar monoterminal). There is a minor difference in the operation of both these applications. The waveform selection is partially rectified.

- After all primary preparation, the waveform partially rectified is selected. The antenna plate is removed from its place and disconnected from the circuit. A straight needle electrode or thicker desiccation electrode is inserted fully inside the handpiece. The power selected is 1, the lowest setting. Moistening

of tissue is not required. The electrode should very finely touch the meat piece for a second or so. The meat tissue will whiten immediately due to dehydration of the superficial cells. This dehydration or desiccation causes superficial necrosis and the lesion peels off or desquamates.

- For demonstration of fulguration, the same electrode is lifted only one millimeter from the meat tissue while the power setting is increased to above 5. When the power is increased above 5, the radio waves jump from the electrode tip to the tissue close by in the form of sparks. These sparks cause the most superficial damage to the meat surface in the form of charring. Here, though the power selected is quite high, the damage is very superficial because of air gap between the electrode tip and meat surface, and the carbon eschar formed by fulguration itself insulates the undersurface from further damage.

Both the electrodessication and electrofulguration applications are very easy to perform and are very useful in dermatologic surgery practice. Many superficial lesions, including verruca plana, milia, skin tags, dermatosis papulosa nigra, molluscum contagiosum, and seborrheic keratosis, are effectively treated using these methods.

Radiovaporization

This is not a separate waveform. It is a function in which the straight needle electrode or fine wire electrode is inserted inside tissue at optimum cutting power using a fully filtered waveform to literally melt the soft tissue inside the bulky mass.

- The power setting is put at 4. The meat piece is held tightly with forceps and the electrode is smoothly inserted inside the bulk of the meat piece. The power is then set to between 3 and 5. The device is started and kept active for some time. The mass is literally seen shrinking due to vaporization of the inside tissue. This is a kind of debulking of tissues.

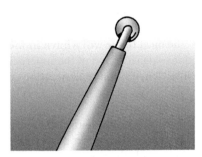

Figure 10.10 Round blade Surgipen.

Sculpting or shaping

This is a specialized artistic technique to literally sculpt or shape the tissue for excellent cosmetic result.

- A fully filtered current is used at a low power of 1 or 2. Either a round loop electrode or a round bladed Surgipen (Figure 10.10) is used.

- Initially, the meat tissue is cut to scoop out some tissue at three to four places with help of a round loop.
- These scars are then shaped perfectly at a power of 1 or 2. The aforementioned electrodes are used to blunt out the edges of these scars.
- The electrode is held at a 45 to 60 degree angle and the scar edges are blunted down. While doing this the sharp edges can be seen getting blunt and the scars resurface well.

This application is a specialized one but a practice on meat will give good confidence.

REFERENCE

1. Pollack SV. Laboratory exercises. In: *Electrosurgery of the Skin*, 1st edition, New York, Churchill Livingstone, 1991, 73–85.

11

Patient assessment and counseling

In dermatology we are faced with numerous skin disorders that cannot be termed as skin diseases but come under the category of cosmetic disfigurement like freckles, moles, keratosis, skin tags, syringoma, milia, and xanthelasma. Patients who approach us with the expectation of getting each and every blemish removed from their skin may be suffering from body dysmorphic disorder. Such patients need to be filtered out or counseled out using rational tactics. But, there are many others who seek removal of many unusual blemishes like every tiny flat mole and who come with unrealistic expectations that everything can be cleansed clear with modern high-tech gadgets like lasers who need to be sincerely counseled without any time constraints. They need to be made aware of the ground reality and limitations of so-called high-tech lasers with the help of photographic record as evidence.

PATIENT CONSULTATION AND ASSESSMENT

The most important meeting between the doctor and the patient is the *consultation*. Patients approach doctors for their opinions about skin problems that are troubling them physically or psychologically. The physical problems can be in the form of a callus, corn, keloid, hypertrophic scar, ingrown toenail, chronic lichenified eczema, prurigo nodularis, or wart. Psychological problems can be due to the cosmetic nature of the skin problem, such as unsightly moles, warts, xanthelasma, skin tags, keratosis, and milia.

Patients who come for removal of a cosmetic skin problem are absolutely healthy. They are very concerned about the lesion spoiling their look and hence demand removal. This patient needs proper timely consultation explaining the procedure in detail with photos and videos. The patient's expectations need to be keenly understood.

All patients are explained the best surgical treatment whether ablative or nonablative, their possible side effects, limitations, and shortcomings with the help of case study photos from a personal library. Postoperative care should also be explained in detail.

The most important points doctors should explain to patients are that brown- or dark-skinned patients most commonly develop postoperative dyschromia or hyperpigmentation at the operated site. Fair-skinned patients commonly develop erythema at the operated site. These lesions almost always clear fully. Scarring is rare in experienced hands.

All the questions and doubts of the patient regarding his/her problem are eventually solved. Unrealistic expectations are removed from the patient's mind.

During the consultation, the operative expenses are explained to the patient.

After all the discussion, the decision is left with the patient. If the patient is convinced, he/she will finalize an operation appointment with the receptionist.

The patient who finalizes the operation appointment is asked to do basic tests of complete blood count (hemogram), bleeding time, clotting time, blood sugar level, Elisa test for HIV, and HBV antigen test. Patients taking blood thinner medicines like aspirin are advised to stop them 2 days prior.

Patients who are posted for nonablative procedures are treated under surface anesthesia (combination of lidocaine and prilocaine in cream). The larger lesions are treated under local anesthesia of lidocaine injection, which is tested prior to operation for sensitivity.

Let us review the ideal profile of the patient who decides to get operated:

- Patient is medically and psychologically stable.
- Clearly defined area of dissatisfaction.
- Realistic expectations.
- Self-motivated.
- Patient is convinced to get desired result.

INFORMED CONSENT

Informed consent is the most important step before any dermatologic surgery begins. The patient is given the informed consent form containing all information about his/her procedure in details for reading and signing to give official permission for the operative procedure.

The informed consent form is the most important document and it should give full details of the operative procedure to be performed. It should contain the proper diagnosis. This form also should contain information about possible side effects, expected results, postoperative care, and a follow-up visit schedule. Detailed patient information should be entered, including name, address, phone number, and signature. Photo documentation is a must and I always get separate permission signatures for this. In case of children under 18 years of age, I get the signature of the parent or guardian.

All informed consent forms should have two important statements (duly signed by the patient):

1. Patient does not have cardiac pacemaker.
2. Local anesthetic lignocaine 2% has been tested and there is no allergic reaction.

This document is of medicolegal value and, hence, should never be ignored however small the surgical procedure may be.

12

Applications

Experience tells you what to do and what not to do; confidence allows you to do it.

Stan Smith

Radiofrequency (RF) surgery is one of the most enterprising tools in dermatologic surgery. I dare to say so because this tool gives you ample scope to not only improvise the surgical methods but also to refine approaches to suit today's need of becoming aesthetically pleasing. Just as technological advances have revolutionized surgery from large incisions to laparoscopic miniaturization, radiofrequency surgery has refined dermatologic surgery from a primitive destructive method to a minimally invasive one.

This and the following three chapters will cover all the applications I have been practicing for the last 18 years when I first started using RF surgery in my clinic. It has been a very interesting period and a very satisfying one as well.

I started RF surgery in May 1999. Earlier I was using electrocautery, cryosurgery, and chemical cautery. As advised, I practiced all the waveforms on meat pieces before starting RF surgery on my first patient. My first patient was a case of single periungual wart on a finger. The patient was prepared for RF surgical excision under local anesthesia in my clinic's procedure room. After giving local anesthesia, I set the machine on "fully filtered current." A round loop electrode was fully inserted inside the handpiece. The power was set at 3. The wart was hydrated with a normal saline solution. I started the procedure by holding the electrode at a right angle to the wart and tried excising the wart. But the electrode dragged and got stuck in warty tissue. With some effort I detached the electrode to restart cutting. I increased the power to 5, but still I could only cut the wart in half and felt the need to increase it

further. So I increased it to 6. To my surprise I cut through the wart within a split second but went farther down into the dermis leading to profuse bleeding. This alarmed me. The wart was fully excised but the last stroke with a slightly higher power caused a deeper cut than expected. Having never done dermatologic surgery with a scalpel in dermatology practice, I was very panicky to see profuse bleeding even though it was of capillary origin. I tried pressure hemostasis and electrocoagulation but that failed to stop it. Since I was not very confident using electrocoagulation, which as I mentioned requires a superficial touch, I finally called my surgeon friend who helped to stop the bleeding with hemostatic solution.

This incident for me was the only one of its kind. The reason I narrate this incident is that as dermatologists we get very panicky on encountering hemorrhage during operation, whereas our surgeon friends deal with it daily.

Radiofrequency surgery technique has changed my career to a flourishing one and this case was the start of it.

My second case was that of a few skin tags around the neck of a young lady. I excised all of them under local anesthesia. I was happy to have the procedure work well, but the patient had a lot of pain during the week until all postoperative wounds fully healed.

The third case was also of skin tags on the neck and in the axillae. I considered desiccating all of them under local anesthesia and followed this to experience a far more comfortable patient till all lesions fully cleared.

Next was a case of multiple warts over a knee. A few were treated using electrocautery by a dermatologist colleague. I would not have had any other opportunity better than this to compare both techniques. The warts treated by electrocautery healed with atrophic scars and the child's mother was very upset. I gave them hope of the newer RF technique for a better outcome and excised them under local anesthesia. The result really proved the superior postoperative outcome of RF surgery.

Cases of milia, molluscum contagiosum, and dermatosis papulosa nigra on the face have been a matter of cosmetic concern. There were no specific references pertaining to each of these indications, but Dr. Sheldon Pollack's book *Electrosurgery of the Skin* has guidelines for using electrodesiccation for various papilloma, skin tags, and so on. On those guidelines, I treated the aforementioned lesions with good results, but there were problems of postinflammatory hyperpigmentation and scarring in some cases.

As new indications came up, with few references in literature, I made some trials and errors to develop new applications based on the finer properties of RF–tissue interactions. Of course, this also required proper knowledge of histopathology of the treated lesions.

I started experimenting with the knowledge of RF–tissue interaction, RF waveforms, all points related to lateral heat dispersion into tissues, and histopathology of various skin lesions to be treated put together to use radiofrequency surgery for the common indications in dermatologic surgery. Once I was confident in using radiofrequency surgery, I further continued experimenting for newer indications.

I soon realized that radiofrequency surgery modality is a versatile method having many indications in dermatologic surgery. It was further realized that this same method can be used for nonsurgical facelifts or skin tightening. Discussion of this indication is beyond the scope of this book.

I classify the applications of radiofrequency surgery broadly as therapeutic and diagnostic.

THERAPEUTIC APPLICATIONS

Therapeutic application of radiofrequency surgery can be further classified into ablative and nonablative:

- *Ablative*—Here, the skin lesions are incised and/or excised using waveforms of either cut or blend with or without electrocoagulation.
- *Nonablative*—Here, the skin lesions are simply desiccated or fulgurated using those respective waveforms (here, though the lesions finally cleared from skin, these lesions are not actually excised or cut during the procedure).

Therapeutic ablative applications (excision) are the among the most common for which radiofrequency surgery is used. Facial and neck lesions amount to more than 50% of the share. People nowadays are very concerned about any and all blemishes on the face, from simple moles to freckles to postacne hyperpigmented spots to warts to new growths to larger moles and cysts. The age group is not the criteria because I see many middle aged and elderly aged ladies and gentlemen walking in my clinic to seek advice for removal of their blemishes on exposed portions of the face and neck that spoil their looks. It is the awareness, medical (fear of skin cancer), or cosmetic concern for which they come prepared to spend.

Therapeutic nonablative applications (desiccation/fulguration) form at least 30% of the total share of radiofrequency surgery patients. These are some of the relatively easier applications but are monetarily rewarding.

DIAGNOSTIC APPLICATIONS

Radiofrequency surgery is one of the best tools for doing a skin biopsy. This is because of its properties of a very thin cut (approximately 10 to 20 microns) and the least lateral tissue damage. Lesions to be removed are planned beforehand for sending them for histopathology either in the form of a small incised portion or in toto.

Lesions to be sent for histopathology are cut using a thin wire electrode or round loop electrode or straight needle electrode, in that order of preference. A fully filtered current or waveform is always used at the lowest effective power. This waveform produces the thinnest cut, hence it is preferred. This is covered in detail in Chapter 16.

13

Specific applications: Radiofrequency commonality

This chapter covers the most common of indications for which radiofrequency (RF) surgery is used and is famous for or is always referred to for. These indications are the bread and butter of a radiofrequency office surgery. Everyone who desires to use radiofrequency surgery in dermatologic surgery or those who have decided to start dermatologic surgery in an office using radiofrequency surgery must be thoroughly acquainted with the minutest details of these indications for the best results.

Refer to Table 13.1 for general guidelines in treating these indications. The power settings are given as per my experience (with the Ellman Surgitron), hence the reader is advised to modify the settings according to individual choice and experience.

Perhaps the most impressive result of radiofrequency surgery is the excision of moles or intradermal nevi, also called melanocytic nevi. However, warts or verrucae are among the most common of all conditions to be treated because of the higher incidence and potential for infection and recurrence.

A stepwise guide to treat the aforementioned common indications are given in the following sections.

MOLES OR INTRADERMAL NEVI OR MELANOCYTIC NEVI

People are very conscious of their appearance today. Any moles on the face and neck bring so many young patients to demand removal. These people feel embarrassed by the moles, thinking they spoil their looks. Or they would like to have a blemish-free face or neck.

Moles are generally removed for cosmetic purposes. Occasionally, patients seek advice for a fast growing mole or new mole appearance fearing possibility of cancer.

Following are some important criteria for selecting moles for excision by radiofrequency surgery:

- Moles should be significantly raised above the skin surface. Only such moles can be easily removed without much scarring as their depth does not extend into the lower dermis.
- Flatter moles can be deeper in depth, hence can cause easy recurrence. Hence, such cases should be counseled against removal.
- All moles must be sent for histopathology as a routine to confirm diagnosis and as a precaution to rule out dysplastic changes of malignancy.

Mole excision technique

See Figures 13.1 to 13.20.

- All preoperative requisites are checked and completed.
- Local anesthetic testing done, informed consent taken, photo documentation completed.
- After sterilization, a lignocaine with adrenaline injection is given underneath the nevus intradermally.
- Wait 5 minutes to start the procedure.
- Electrode choice is almost always round loop.

Table 13.1 Ready reckoner for common applications

Skin lesion	Waveform	Electrode	Power*
Moles or melanocytic nevus	RFE	L	3–5
Verruca vulgaris	RFE/RFB	L/T	3–5
Verruca plana	RFD	S/D	1–2
Skin tags	RFE/RFB	S/L	3–5
Skin tags	RFD	S/D	1–2
Dermatosis papulosa nigra	RFD	S	1
Milia	RFD	S	1
Corns/calluses	RFE/RFB	S and L/T	3–8
Keratoses	RFE	L	3–4
Sebaceous cysts	RFE	TW/S	3–4

Note: D, broad needle electrode for desiccation and fulguration; L, round loop electrode; RFB, radiofrequency blend waveform; RFD, radiofrequency desiccation waveform; RFE, radiofrequency excision (cut) waveform; S, straight needle electrode; T, triangular electrode; TW, thin wire electrode.
* Power settings vary with the equipment used.

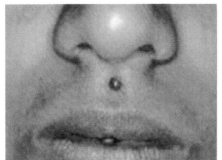
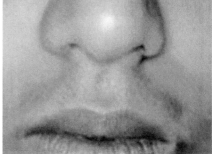

Figure 13.1 Excellent removal of mole without residual scar. (From Biju Vasudevan, *Procedural Dermatosurgery, A Step by Step Approach*, Jaypee Brothers Medical Book Publishers Pvt. Ltd., 2018.)

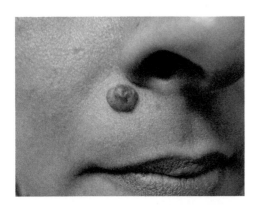
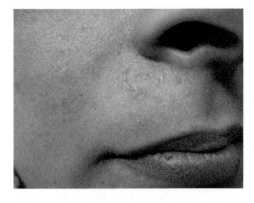

Figure 13.2 Mole before removal.

Figure 13.3 Immediately after mole excision (excellent and clean postoperative wound).

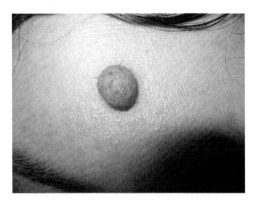

Figure 13.4 Mole before removal.

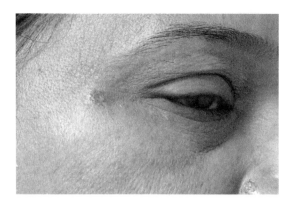

Figure 13.7 Immediately after mole excision.

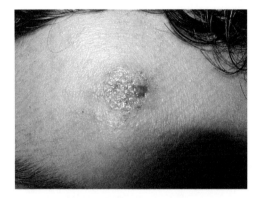

Figure 13.5 Immediately after mole excision (excellent and clean postoperative wound).

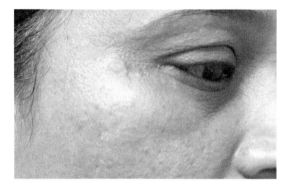

Figure 13.8 Two weeks after mole excision.

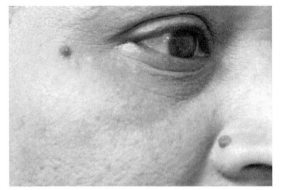

Figure 13.6 Two moles before excision.

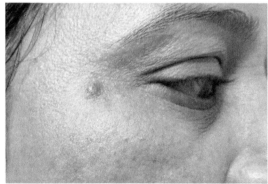

Figure 13.9 One month after mole excision.

- The waveform is always cut or fully filtered.
- Power is set to 3 and the handpiece containing the electrode is held at a right angle or perpendicular to the skin surface.
- A rough assessment is made to confirm whether the power selected is optimum to make a microsmooth incision.

- Once the optimum power is set, the first aim is to remove a small piece or in toto of the skin lesion to be sent for histopathology. This requires operative experience and skill to take a biopsy piece in one stroke. Holding and slightly stretching the adjoining skin between the index finger and thumb of the inactive

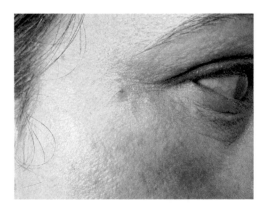

Figure 13.10 One year after mole excision, mild recurrence seen near right eye.

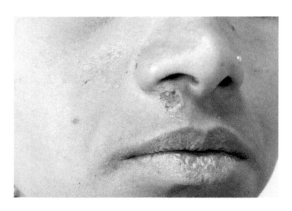

Figure 13.13 Immediately after mole excision (black mole tissue persists in deeper skin layer).

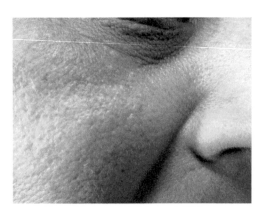

Figure 13.11 One year after mole excision (no recurrence on nostril), no scar seen.

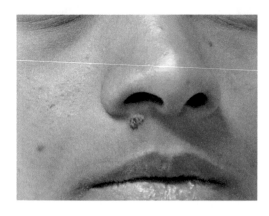

Figure 13.14 Recurrence after 2 months.

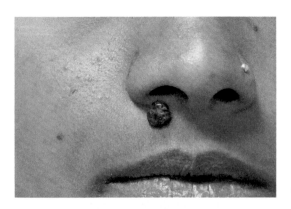

Figure 13.12 Mole near right nostril.

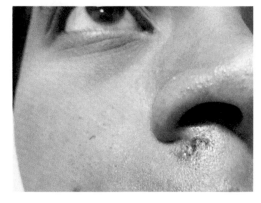

Figure 13.15 Immediately after second excision. If mole tissue still persists, it will require removal by a cosmetic surgeon.

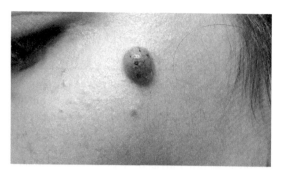

Figure 13.16 Mole on left cheek.

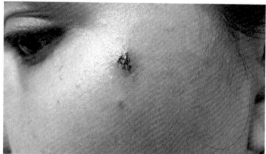

Figure 13.19 Two months after mole excision shows significant recurrence.

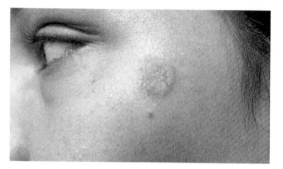

Figure 13.17 Mole on left cheek immediately after excision.

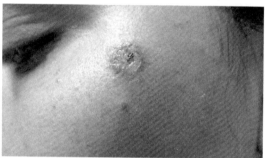

Figure 13.20 Mole excised again.

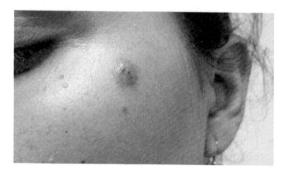

Figure 13.18 One month after mole excision shows recurrence.

hand, the bulk of the mole tissue is excised in a single stroke. The excised mole tissue is put in formol saline for histopathology.

- The rest of the mole tissue is trimmed with the shave excision method until all remnants of mole tissue have cleared.

- If in case after reaching the level of the papillary dermis the mole tissue is still visible in some portion, especially in the center, it is desirable to leave it as it is to prevent scarring. The patient is shown the condition on-table and explained the possibility of scarring if efforts are made to remove deeper mole tissue, and that it is desirable to wait and watch for 6 to 8 weeks to see if it regrows. In that case, if the patient is still demanding to remove it, this will require deeper excision leading to scarring.
- Once the mole tissue is excised, pressure hemostasis is employed with saline-soaked gauze for 5 minutes, which usually stops the capillary bleeding. I prefer not to use electrocoagulation unless required.
- The most important job of blending is done now to blend the open wound tissue with the adjoining epidermis of intact skin with the same electrode at a lower power of 1 or 2 only.

The electrode is kept at a right angle or tilted to achieve this result. Good experience is required to do this skillfully. It is a very critical step for superior cosmetic results.

- A postoperative photograph is taken.
- The wound is dressed with antibiotic ointment.
- Postoperative care is explained and medicines prescribed (refer to Chapter 17).

Follow-up

- All patients are advised to come for a follow-up visit after one week.
- Wound healing is closely observed (whether complete or not).
- If wound has fully healed, the patient is advised to revisit after 2 weeks.
- In the next visit, the healed wound is closely observed for the start of hyperpigmentation or erythema in the healed scar.
- Any signs of hyperpigmentation is treated with standard bleaching creams for 2 to 4 weeks until it clears.
- Patient is later called at the end of one month approximately to see the response to bleaching creams to find out whether there are any early signs of recurrence of the mole.
- If there is no recurrence at the end of 8 weeks after surgery, it is unlikely to recur.
- Some patients (<10%) show recurrence in the form of a small, black-colored, dotlike spot or frank mole recurrence.
- Decision about repeat excision is taken at the end of 6 to 8 weeks.
- The recurrent mole is always reexcised under local anesthesia in a similar fashion but with a slightly deeper excision to prevent further recurrence. The patient is well informed beforehand about a deep excision and the possibility of a superficial scar later.
- A small dotlike clump of melanocytes may not increase in size and may be left untreated as the dot is hardly seen. This position can remain stable for years.
- Any superficial scar resulting from excision can be effectively resurfaced using a special technique of radiofrequency for scar resurfacing later.
- Any postoperative hyperpigmentation or erythema or superficial scar becomes virtually invisible after 2 months as the collagen remodeling is completed.

WARTS (VERRUCA PLANA, VERRUCA VULGARIS, DIGITATE, OR FILIFORM WARTS)

Warts, or verrucae, are some of the most common indications for RF surgery. These occur in all age groups and there is no effective oral treatment for it. They affect the skin of any area from the scalp to the soles. Being of viral origin with the potential to spread to other areas or to other people, urgent removal remains the best option. Being symptomless, patients commonly neglect them until the warts affect some area on the face or start causing discomfort or pain, especially the periungual and the plantar ones. Patients usually try all kinds of alternate therapies such as home remedies or advertised products, or alternative medicines like homeopathy or herbal medicine before considering RF surgery.

Approach to warts treatment

- Always take a detailed history of patients and examine them thoroughly to have a proper idea of the number of warts and their distribution on the body.
- Sometimes only a few warts are present with the rest likely to be microscopic and thus invisible, whereas sometimes there could be numerous warts spread all over the body.
- Patient's immune status should be assessed and may have to be investigated if in doubt.
- If there are a few on the face, a treatment has to be planned that will give the best cosmetic result.
- If the warts are on the scalp, the whole area must be thoroughly examined because this and beard areas are notorious for recurrence and warts can be hidden in hairy areas.
- If the number of warts is in the dozens, plan treatment in two to three sessions at intervals of 1 to 2 weeks.
- If plantar warts are multiple, again all cannot be treated in one session.
- Periungual, plantar, and scalp warts are likely to bleed more.
- Sometimes skin warts are seen spread over mucosal areas such as nasal, oral, and genital areas. These require a different approach (see later).

Counseling

- Patients approaching for warts treatment should be informed that this is a viral infection by human papilloma virus and can spread to other areas and to other persons through direct contact and indirect contact (fomites or shared articles). There is no documented full-proof oral treatment. Hence, prevention is very important even if the treatment is given.
- In spite of the best treatment given, chances of recurrence are always there because either the new microscopic lesions have grown, or some old lesions have recurred, or patient's immunity is less against them.
- There are some other methods I employ to improve immunity like giving oral Levamisol.
- In my experience the recurrence gradually regresses over a period of a few months.

Wart removal technique

EXCISION

See Figures 13.21 to 13.27.

- Excision is always under local anesthesia, which is tested prior as before.
- Selection is always done beforehand, explained to patients, informed consent signed, and preoperative photography done.
- If there are multiple warts on the face and elsewhere, I prefer not to excise all, because excision leads to open wounds, which are more painful and likely to get infected. Here, I always combine excision with desiccation for

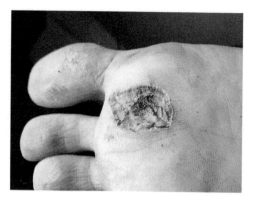

Figure 13.22 Plantar wart clean excision.

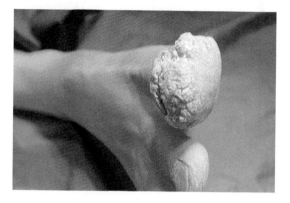

Figure 13.23 Periungual and subungual warts.

better patient tolerance and comfort as well as to prevent infection.

- I prefer desiccation for facial lesions to prevent facial wounding, dyschromia, chances of sepsis, and scarring unless there are only one to two warts.
- All warts are marked before giving a lignocaine with adrenaline injection underneath. Periungual areas are injected with lignocaine (plain).
- A round loop electrode or triangular electrode is used for excision.
- Usually the blend or cut + coagulation waveform is selected.
- The power is usually 3 to 10 depending upon the thickness of the wart.
- Simultaneous coagulation helps bloodless cutting. This is better for warts on the scalp, palms, soles, or periungual areas.
- Where the cosmetic end result is important, as on the face and neck, I prefer using a cut

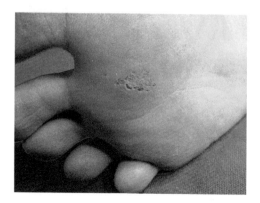

Figure 13.21 Plantar wart.

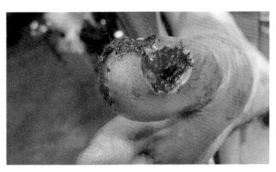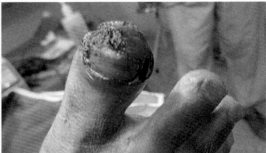

Figure 13.24 Periungual and subungual warts clean excision.

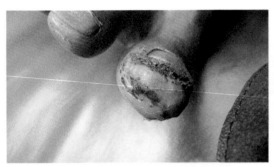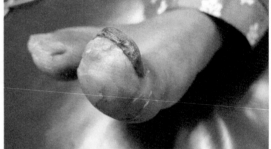

Figure 13.25 Very good complete healing after warts excision.

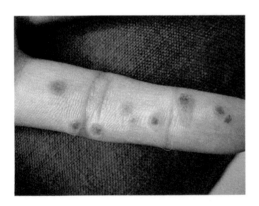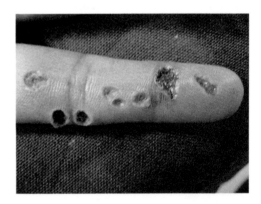

Figure 13.26 Multiple finger warts.

Figure 13.27 Multiple finger warts completely excised.

or fully filtered waveform. Here, a power of 3 to 5 is usually used, which gives superior excision. Some bleeding is expected which can be arrested with pressure hemostasis. Electrocoagulation is used only if bleeding continues even after pressure hemostasis.

- For excising periungual warts, a digital block with a lignocaine injection (plain) is given.
- Some periungual warts may have extended subungually. Here, cutting the nail over the subungual warty portion will facilitate excision.

- All warts must be excised thoroughly, deep enough to excise all the visible warty tissue and the border of the excision extending at least 2 mm surrounding the wart border to prevent recurrence.
- In all excisions for warts, except those on the face, I prefer using electrocoagulation with a ball electrode performing soft coagulation at a power of 5 or 6. I follow this because electro-coagulation destroys tissue with more lateral tissue heat dispersion. This causes charring or carbonization of tissues leading to necrosis in areas deeper and away from borders of the wart. This step, in my experience, helps prevent recurrence.
- Dressing and postoperative care are the same as described earlier and covered in Chapter 17.

DESICCATION

- I prefer using this method for facial and neck warts, especially when they are many in number and small in size.
- Verruca plana or plane warts are very common on the face. Desiccation is very good for such lesions.
- I treat verruca plana under surface anesthesia (topical lidocaine and prilocaine).
- For bigger warts (verruca vulgaris), I prefer desiccating them under local anesthesia.
- After preliminary preparation and anesthesia given, the machine is turned on.
- I use a straight needle or broad needle electrode.
- Waveform selection is done for desiccation.
- Power is set to 1 or 2, and there is no antenna plate.
- The electrode is superficially touched (a fine touch) just for a second or so until the wart whitens (dehydration). Whitening or dehydration of warts leads to wart necrosis and scab formation. This dead warty tissue separates or gets peeled off within a week maximum.
- This method is very fast and good for numerous small warts.
- This method is of no use for large warts, palmoplantar warts, or scalp warts.
- Postoperative care is given in Chapter 17.

Follow-up

- All patients should be followed up for a minimum of 3 months.
- Any postoperative dyschromia or scars are further treated.
- Recurrence is treated as mentioned earlier.

SKIN TAGS

Skin tags or acrochordons are very common. These are among the least reported skin problems because they are symptomless. Skin tags affect many areas of the body, namely, the face, neck, axillae, back, abdomen, thighs, and buttocks. Patients normally avoid taking treatment for these unless required, especially when they affect exposed areas of the face and neck, or when they cause pain or difficulty in wearing clothes and ornaments or making movements. Patients also avoid removal of these because they feel some surgery will be required.

Removal techniques

EXCISION

- After completing all primary preparations, the skin tags are anesthetized with a lignocaine with adrenaline injection using an insulin syringe. I prefer an insulin syringe because the needle is 27 gauge and thus injection pain is less.
- A straight needle electrode or round loop electrode is selected.
- A cut or blend waveform is selected and the machine is turned on.
- The power set to 3 to 5 is preferred.
- The skin tag is held with toothed forceps and the electrode is just pushed through at the base to excise it in one stroke.
- The round loop electrode may be pushed around the skin tag to its base, which is then held with forceps, and the electrode is then only pulled through to excise the tag in one stroke. For this method it is best to keep the power set to 4 or 5 instead of a lower power and finding the electrode stuck in the tissue of the tag. I usually do not prefer this method because sometimes blindly one may cut a bit deeper while sliding the electrode through the tag from the opposite side towards towards oneself. I prefer excising it by just holding it with

forceps and cutting through with a straight needle or round loop electrode. The round loop electrode is preferable when working over the face and neck because it is very thin.

- If the cut waveform is used, there could be bleeding.
- Electrocoagulation may be used for hemostasis if pressure doesn't work.
- Usually no dressing is needed. The wound heals in a week's time.
- Postoperative care remains the same.

DESICCATION

See Figure 13.28.

- Desiccation is best for all small skin tags.
- Surface anesthesia (a topical cream containing lidocaine and prilocaine) is applied for a minimum of 45 minutes before the procedure.
- Primary preparations are completed as before.
- A straight needle electrode or broad needle electrode is selected.
- The rest of the steps remain the same as described earlier for warts.
- All the treated skin tags whiten due to dehydration, shrink in size immediately, become necrosed, then fall off within a week.
- This method is best for multiple small skin tags. I have treated more than 25 to 30 in one session.
- There is mild inflammation of adjoining skin at each skin tag base, which subsides in 1 hour.

- I prefer using the straight needle electrode. I use the broad needle electrode for larger skin tags.

DERMATOSIS PAPULOSA NIGRA (DPN)

Dermatosis papulosa nigra, a benign cutaneous unsightly condition, is very common in Indians. Nowadays it is very commonly reported by patients who demand removal. Many patients have plenty of them affecting the face and neck. Commonly ladies seek removal. These lesions are very superficial and hence the desiccation method is best.

Desiccation

The primary steps and surface anesthesia particulars remain the same as given earlier (see Warts section).

- The waveform of electrodessication is selected. The antenna plate is not connected.
- The straight needle electrode is my choice.
- Power of 1 is best.
- These lesions are 1 to 5 mm and very superficial, so each lesion is just finely touched with the electrode tip for just a second until it whitens due to dehydration.
- As with desiccation, all lesions are left to fall off automatically in a week's time.

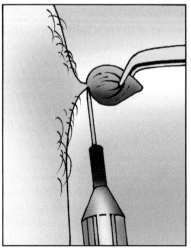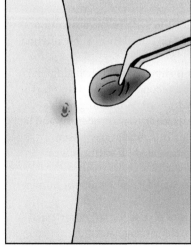

Figure 13.28 Excision of pedunculated skin tag.

- There will be mild inflammation around each lesion, which will subside in an hour.
- There is mild burning pain after the procedure.
- I prefer using the cut mode if lesions are very tiny, because of minimum lateral heat dispersion, and power is kept at 1. Lesions are left to fall off.
- I do not prefer a thin wire electrode because it is very fine and each DPN lesion may require more than one fine contact or a longer contact time, increasing the possibility of side effects.

MILIA

These tiny, skin-colored cystic lesions very commonly affect the cheeks, eyelids, and nose. These lesions spoil the appearance of a person. Milia are very common in all age groups. People 20 to 50 years of age are troubled due to their unsightly nature. Treatment is always for cosmetic purpose.

Desiccation

- All the basic steps remain the same. Surface anesthesia is as usual.
- The electrodessication waveform is selected.
- I use the cut mode, especially on tiny milia on the eyelids.
- All other observations remain the same.
- Treated milia will automatically clear off to give a very clean looking face.
- The straight needle electrode is preferred.
- Power is mentioned in Table 13.1.

CORNS AND CALLUSES

Corns and calluses are quite common in dermatology practice. But, many people do approach their family physicians or general surgeons. Many try all sorts of home remedies before approaching a dermatologist. Some have experienced recurrence after surgical removal. Removing corns and calluses is an easy task overall. Prevention of recurrence is a tough task. Besides the routine causes for corns and calluses there are few important causes that require special mention here. In dermatology, I have seen a number of patients who have neuropathy due to either diabetes, leprosy, alcohol, or other causes developing these. In these patients especially, the postoperative wound care and prevention of recurrence is extremely important.

A casual approach for wound healing here will lead to complications as well. Hence, I have highlighted the postoperative wound care in detail. I prefer moistening or hydration for all lesions before excision.

Excision

See Figures 13.29 and 13.30.

- All the basic steps for excision remain the same.
- Lignocaine with adrenaline is filled in a 5 ml disposable syringe and given underneath the selected corn or callus.
- Wait for 5 minutes minimum.
- The cut or blend waveform is selected.
- A straight needle, round loop or triangular electrode, and ball electrode are kept ready.

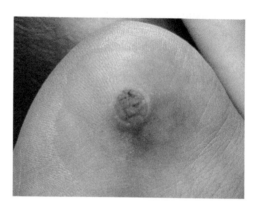

Figure 13.29 Corn wart.

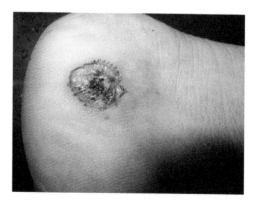

Figure 13.30 Corn wart excision (clean postoperative wound).

- The power selected should be 3 or 4 minimum for the cut mode and at least two levels higher more for the blend mode.
- Initially, with the straight needle electrode I mark the border of any corn or callus. After this step, I increase the power by one or two to deepen the marked border from one side. I later hold this cut edge with toothed forceps and go on excising the whole corn or callus. The whole corn or callus is excised and shown to the patient.
- The electrode is changed to round loop or triangular.
- The appearance as well as tactile feel gives a good idea of the remnants of the corn/callus and are thus excised.
- Bleeding is arrested using electrocoagulation.
- I generally take a slightly larger incision around the corn or callus beyond the marked border to prevent recurrence.
- I always keenly observe the hard tissue and even palpate it to confirm complete removal.
- The postoperative wound is always very clean. This advantage is of immense importance for neuropathy patients.
- Postoperative care is very important to prevent recurrence.

Postoperative care and follow-up

- Postoperatively, wound care should be as usual with change of dressing daily.
- Oral antibiotic is given for 7 to 10 days.
- Pain-relieving medicines are given for 2 to 3 days and are optional.
- I always advise patients to do the dressing in the clinic and not at home.
- Wound sepsis has to be avoided.
- Normal walking for daily routine is allowed.
- Excess standing and walking must be avoided until the wound is healed, which takes 10 to 15 days.
- Even after wound healing, the collagen remodeling activity continues for more than a month, hence walking as an exercise must be avoided for at least one month. Premature excess walking or standing puts extra pressure on newly formed scar and predisposes it to hypertrophy and recurrence.

- Also, barefoot walking and standing must be avoided for the same reason. Soft footwear with a soft insole is preferable to prevent recurrence.
- If the aforementioned precautions and care is strictly followed, recurrence is unlikely.

KERATOSES (SEBORRHEIC AND ACTINIC)

Keratoses are superficial benign growths occurring commonly over the face, scalp, chest, abdomen, back, and shoulders. These are brown or black, slightly raised over the skin surface, and may have a verrucous or warty surface. They also have a waxy and stuck-on appearance. They could be small sized (1–3 mm) or larger (up to 1 cm or more). They are totally symptomless. Patients approach many times for cosmetic reasons or occasionally out of fear of malignancy if suddenly found. Actinic keratosis appears commonly on fair skin over sun-exposed areas like the face, bald scalp, and forearms. The possibility of melanoma and basal cell carcinoma should always be kept in mind while excising these lesions and hence excised lesions should be sent for histopathology.

Excision

See Figures 13.31 to 13.45.

- All primary preparation as mentioned earlier.
- A local anesthetic of lignocaine with adrenaline is injected underneath the lesion.
- The loop electrode is preferred.

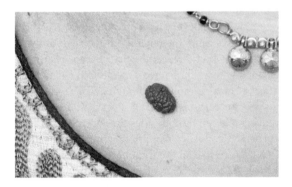

Figure 13.31 Seborrheic keratosis on chest.

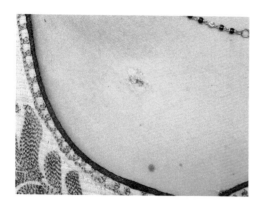

Figure 13.32 Seborrheic keratosis excised completely.

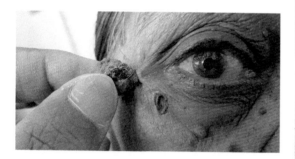

Figure 13.33 Seborrheic keratosis (pedunculated) near right eye.

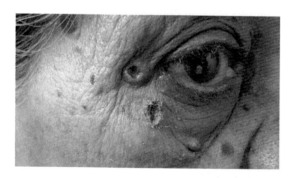

Figure 13.34 Hemostasis was done using electrocoagulation to remove seborrheic keratosis (pedunculated) near right eye.

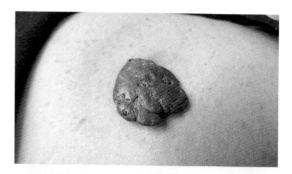

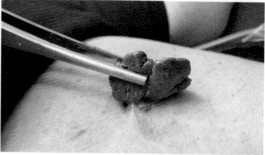

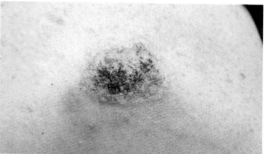

Figure 13.35 Large pedunculated seborrhoeic keratosis over back excised cleanly (hemostasis done with electrocoagulation).

- A cut waveform is selected with a power of 3 or 4.
- Thickened verrucous lesions may require a power of 5 or 6.
- Smaller lesions can be excised in a single stroke and sent for histopathology, but for larger lesions of 1 cm size, an incision biopsy of part of the lesion is taken.
- Later, the lesion is very finely cleared from the skin surface using fine paintbrush-like or "portrait-shading" strokes.

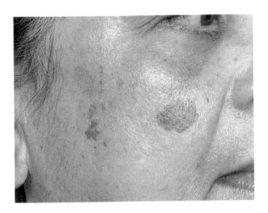

Figure 13.36 Actinic keratosis on right cheek.

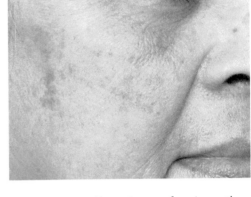

Figure 13.38 Excellent picture after 6 months (negligible scarring).

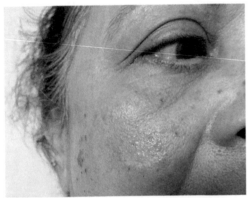

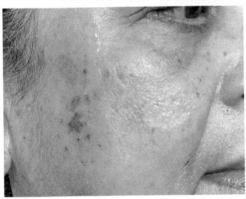

Figure 13.37 Immediately after excision (very nice and clean postoperative wound, not much bleeding, pressure hemostasis done).

- A very steady hand is essential for such strokes not to allow a deeper cut.
- With each stroke, one will observe the brown-black pigmented remains of keratosis getting

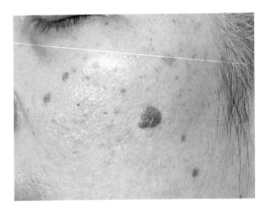

Figure 13.39 Actinic keratosis and dermatosis papulosa nigra on right cheek.

cleared and the surface appearing clean without much of bleeding.
- Once the full lesion is removed, the edges are blended with the adjoining normal skin at a power of 1. This is a very critical task for best results.
- All excised lesions appear like superficial abrasions and hence dressing is not required generally unless the wound is large or in body folds.
- All heal in a week's time.
- Some small keratoses can be treated using the desiccation method; biopsy cannot be taken if desiccation only is used.
- Postoperative care is as usual.

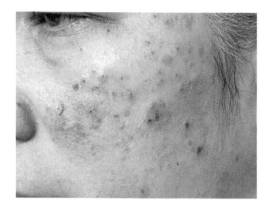

Figure 13.40 Larger actinic keratosis excised (clean excision). Small actinic keratosis and dermatosis papulosa nigra are electrodesiccated under surface anesthesia.

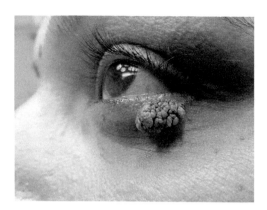

Figure 13.43 Large seborrheic keratosis on left lower eyelid in close proximity to eyelashes.

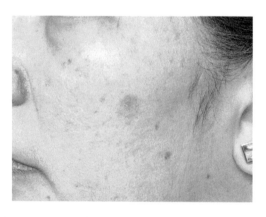

Figure 13.41 Mild postoperative erythema (fair skin) at the end of 2 months.

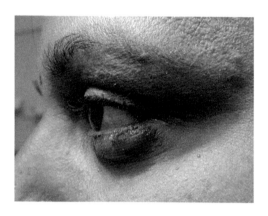

Figure 13.44 Very clean excision of large seborrheic keratosis was done using pressure hemostasis.

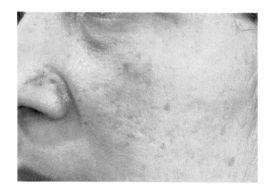

Figure 13.42 No scarring after 6 months.

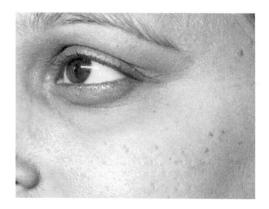

Figure 13.45 No scarring 2 months later.

SEBACEOUS CYSTS

Sebaceous cysts are quite commonly seen in practice. Being harmless, patients usually do not bother to treat them unless infected. These are commonly seen on the scalp, face, neck, chest, and back. They can be removed by two methods explained next. See Figures 13.46 to 13.49.

Routine surgical method

- All primary preparations are as usual.
- A lignocaine with adrenaline injection is given between the superficial skin and cyst wall with a 27 or 30 gauge needle to anesthetize.
- A thin wire electrode is selected.
- The cut waveform is selected.
- Power should only be 2 to 4.
- An elliptical incision is made around the cyst.
- The cyst is dissected out from the tissue adhesions and pulled out with toothed forceps and excised with a thin wire electrode.
- There is hardly any bleeding.

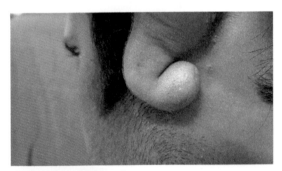

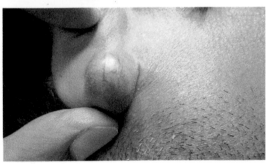

Figure 13.46 Sebaceous cyst.

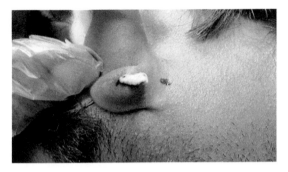

Figure 13.47 Fine and very small cut made with a thin wire electrode on a sebaceous cyst. The sebum is expressed out.

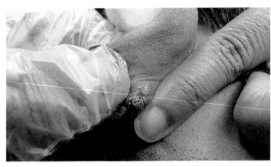

Figure 13.48 Cyst wall expressed out, pulled out with forceps, then cut.

- The edges of the incision are then sutured with interrupted Prolene sutures.
- The cyst is sent for histopathology.

Alternate method

- My preferred method.
- This is very good routinely for not only small cysts but also larger ones.
- Here, after anesthetizing, a very fine incision (nick) of 2 to 4 mm length, only slightly deeper into the cyst wall, is made using a thin wire electrode.
- Sometimes, the fine nick will just be able to let the small cyst pop out through it to be easily enucleated.
- Otherwise, the bisected cyst will open releasing the contents, which should then be squeezed

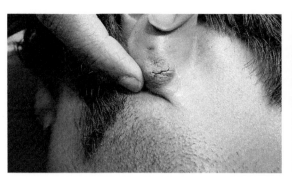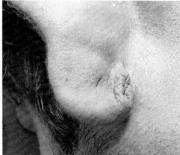

Figure 13.49 Cut edges approximated using tissue glue.

out with lateral pressure. The contents are very foul smelling and one should be careful while squeezing out the contents as that can soil the clothes.

- Once all the contents are expressed out, the cyst wall is pulled out with toothed forceps and cut.
- Usually there is not much bleeding.

- The small hole or opening made with a thin wire electrode is so small that it can be left without suturing to heal by secondary intention.
- Here, the parameters related to waveform, electrode, and power are the same as given in the routine surgical method.

14

Expanding the applications of radiofrequency dermatologic surgery

Radiofrequency (RF) surgery is a versatile tool. With experience you will be able to expand the applications of radiofrequency surgery by making full use of the set of electrodes provided with the equipment by the manufacturer. As you work more with the machine, you can develop more applications taking into account the histopathology of skin conditions, the electrodes, the waveforms, and power. In all applications, the art of the use of electrodes will always make a great difference as far as the cosmetic outcome is concerned.

Table 14.1 contains some of the common applications that I later developed. In addition to applications in Table 14.1, there are few more that though not commonly done still show the versatility of radiofrequency surgery. Please refer to Table 14.2 for details.

I will be touching upon a few selected applications to highlight the practical points while dealing with them.

MOLLUSCUM CONTAGIOSUM

Molluscum contagiosum is a very common viral infection that needs urgent treatment because of its potential to spread to other areas. Though commonly seen in children, its incidence in adults has significantly increased. Nowadays, we encounter many cases of "giant" molluscum in adults and occasionally in children as well. In children, the face and neck are very commonly affected, whereas the face and neck are very commonly affected, whereas in adults, the face, genitals, and groins are commonly affected. See Figures 14.1 to 14.4.

- All molluscum lesions are best treated using the desiccation method.
- I prefer a straight needle electrode or even a thin wire electrode for tiny and small lesions on a child's face. A broad needle electrode may be used in bigger lesions.
- As described earlier, desiccation whitens the lesions due to dehydration and the molluscum body also is coagulated and necrosed due to heat generated. There is no need to enucleate a molluscum body; it gets necrosed and blends with the scab of desiccation to peel off within a week.
- Large or giant molluscum are best excised under local anesthesia.
- Multiple molluscum on the face, genitals, and groin are best treated under surface or topical anesthesia.
- Multiple molluscum in children can be treated in a single session in the operation theater under short duration general anesthesia; done as a "daycare" procedure.
- Immune status needs to be investigated in case of multiple molluscum in adults, especially to rule out HIV infection.
- All treated patients must be followed up for recurrence and reinfection, which is very common, and counseling must be done beforehand to emphasize this.
- Chances of scarring are negligible.

Table 14.1 Ready reckoner for common applications

Skin lesion	Waveform	Electrode	Power
Molluscum contagiosum	RFD	S/B	1–2
Syringoma	RFD	S/B	1
Senile comedones	RFD	S/B	1
Closed comedones (whiteheads)	RFD/RFE	S	1
Xanthelasma	RFD	S	1
Cherry angioma	RFD/RFC	S/B	1
Earlobe repair	RFE	TW	3
Mucocele	RFB	S/L	3–4
Capillary hemangioma	RFB and RFC	L and B	3–6
Pyogenic granuloma	RFB and RFC	L and B	3–6
Trichoepithelioma	RFE	L	3–4
Neurofibroma	RFE	L	3–4
Cutaneous horns	RFE	S/L	3–4
Keratoacanthoma	RFE	L	3–4
Freckles	RFE	S	1
Mucosal lesions (warts, fibroma, etc.)	RFE/RFB	L/T	3–5
	RFD	S/D	1–2

Notes: RFE, radiofrequency excision (cut) waveform; RFB, radiofrequency blend waveform; RFD, radiofrequency desiccation waveform; RFC, radiofrequency coagulation waveform; S, straight needle electrode; L, round loop electrode; T, triangular electrode; B, ball electrode TW, thin wire electrode; D, broad needle electrode.

Table 14.2 Ready reckoner for genital and other uncommon lesions

Skin lesion	Waveform	Electrode	Power
Hypertrophic scar/keloid	RFE/RFB	S and L/T	3–8
	RFC	B	5–10
Condyloma acuminata	RFE/RFB	L/T	3–4
	RFD	S/D	1–2
Genital lesions	RFE/RFB	L/T	3–4
	RFD	S/D	1–2
Periungual and subungual lesions	RFB	S and L	3–8
	RFC	B	6–10
Ingrown toenail	RFC	M	5–6
Rhinophyma	RFE	L	3–5
Gray facial hair	RFC	H	1
Chronic lichenified eczema	RFB	L	3–6
Prurigo nodularis	RFB	L	3–6
Hypertrophic lichen planus	RFB	L/T	3–6
Any papular or nodular lesion of unknown etiology	RFE/RFB	L/T	3–6
Telangiectasia	RFC	STE	1
Basal cell carcinoma	RFE/RFB	L	3–6

Notes: RFE, radiofrequency excision (cut) waveform; RFB, radiofrequency blend waveform; RFD, radiofrequency desiccation waveform; RFC, radiofrequency coagulation waveform; S, straight needle electrode; L, round loop electrode; T, triangular electrode; B, ball electrode; M, matrixectomy electrode; H, hair-removing electrode (insulated), three sizes; STE, special telangiectasia electrode TW, thin wire electrode; D, broad needle electrode.

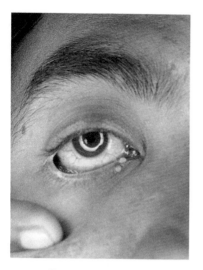

Figure 14.1 Molluscum contagiosum near eye.

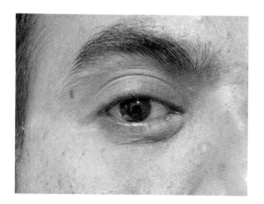

Figure 14.2 Molluscum contagiosum near eye were electrodesiccated under local anesthesia.

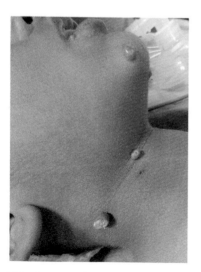

Figure 14.3 Giant molluscum contagiosum over neck and chin in a child.

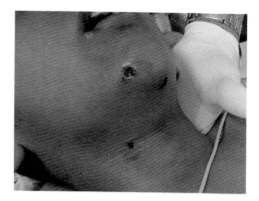

Figure 14.4 Clean excision of giant molluscum contagiosum was done under short general anesthesia in operation theater.

SYRINGOMAS

Syringomas are small superficial lesions arising from the eccrine glands and they commonly present around the eyes causing cosmetic disfigurement. See Figures 14.5 to 14.7.

- Syringomas are difficult to treat in one session.
- I treat multiple lesions in two to four sessions at fortnightly intervals.
- Only soft-touch desiccation should be done without overlap.
- Overzealous treatment may lead to hypo- or hyperpigmented scarring.
- Some lesions may not respond in spite of proper treatment.
- Recurrence is always possible, so patients should be aware of that.

SENILE COMEDONES

Senile comedones are very superficial lesions and commonly grouped over the nose, eyelids, and cheeks. The blackheads can be easily expressed out with a comedone expressor, but recur quickly. See Figures 14.8 and 14.9.

- Single session treatment.
- Surface or local anesthesia.
- Soft touch desiccation is best.
- All lesions will fall off within one week.
- Generally no possibility of scarring.

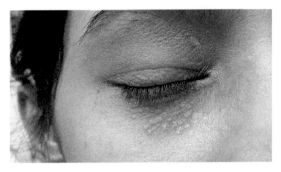
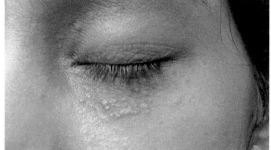

Figure 14.5 Syringoma.

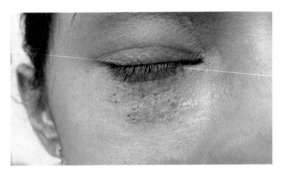
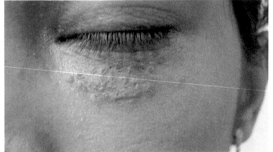

Figure 14.6 Immediately after electrodessication of syringoma.

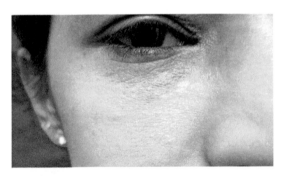
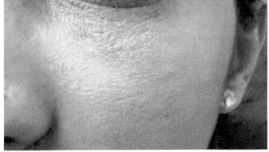

Figure 14.7 Two months after electrodessication of syringoma (almost cleared).

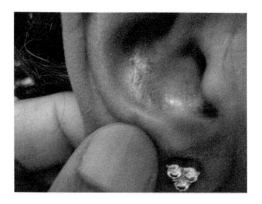

Figure 14.8 Senile comedones in ear.

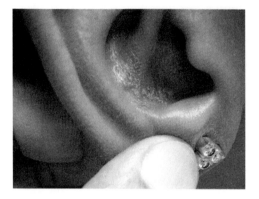

Figure 14.9 Senile comedones immediately after electrodessication.

CLOSED COMEDONES

Some patients of acne have numerous closed comedones on the face. These lesions can be stubborn to applications of topical retinoid and chemical peels. These lesions cannot be expressed out.

- These lesions respond very nicely to the radio-frequency method.
- It is advisable to use the cut waveform, thin wire electrode, with a power of 1 for very tiny

lesions to minimize lateral heat damage on the face.
- Overall, use of a straight needle electrode at a power of 1 with a desiccation waveform is best with very soft touch treatment.
- I prefer treating multiple lesions in two sessions spaced at a fortnight interval.
- All lesions clear within a week. There could be dyschromia but clears eventually with bleaching creams.

XANTHELASMA

Xanthelasma lesions affect the upper and lower eyelids and are unsightly. All patients are advised to get a lipid profile done before surgery to find out if they have deranged lipids like cholesterol. This is not a rule. See Figures 14.10 and 14.11.

- The electrodessication method works out best here, because the lesions are very superficial and the eyelid skin is very thin.
- I sometimes use the cut waveform at a power of 1 to have the least lateral tissue thermal damage to critically thin eyelid skin. The straight needle electrode is best.

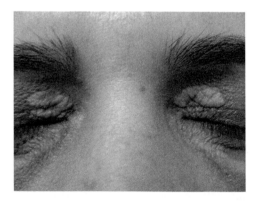

Figure 14.10 Xanthelasma on upper eyelids.

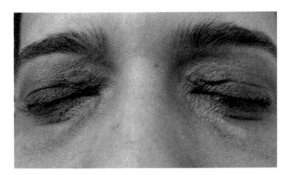

Figure 14.11 Xanthelasma immediately after treatment using electrodessication or electrosection at power 1.

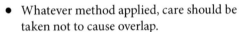

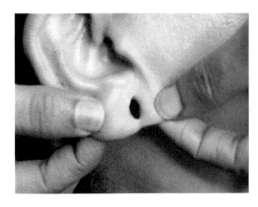

Figure 14.12 Ear lobe before treatment.

- Whatever method applied, care should be taken not to cause overlap.
- Larger lesions are treated in more than one session at fortnightly intervals.

CHERRY ANGIOMAS

Nowadays, many patients demand removal of cherry angiomas. These are distributed over the arms, trunk, and face, and are small (1–5 mm). These are benign growths from skin capillaries. Treatment is purely for cosmetic reasons.

- Waveforms of electrodessication or electrocoagulation can be used at a power of 1.
- A ball electrode can coagulate the lesion fully within a second.
- I use a straight needle electrode for smaller lesions.
- The scab thus formed clears off within a week.
- Scarring is unlikely.

EARLOBE REPAIR

Demand for earlobe repair has increased in all age groups with the increasing use of fashionable ear ornaments. There could be incomplete (partial), complete, or multiple tears. See Figures 14.12 to 14.16.

- Whatever may be the tear, the torn edges are refreshed or finely excised with a thin wire electrode at a power of 3 or 4 using a cut waveform.
- There is usually no bleeding.
- Partial tears having an area less than half the diameter of the earlobe can then be safely stuck

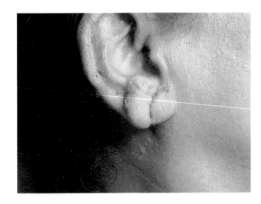

Figure 14.13 Ear lobe repair done using tissue glue.

using cyanoacrylate tissue glue after properly approximating the edges. Aftercare only stresses upon avoiding pressure or traction on the treated side for one week minimum. This method is generally the simplest and result-oriented as well.
- Longer tears or complete tears or multiple tears should be sutured after finely excising edges for best results.
- All procedures are performed under local anesthesia.

MUCOCELES (SUBMUCOUS CYSTS)

Mucoceles are quite common. These can be easily excised using RF under local anesthesia.

- After anesthetizing the lesion, chalazion forceps is used to firmly hold the lesion.

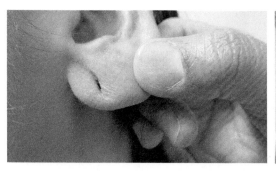

Figure 14.14 Ear lobe front and back (before treatment).

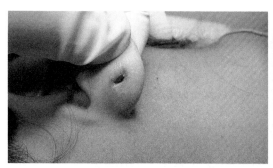

Figure 14.15 Edges freshened up using thin wire electrode under local anesthesia (front and back).

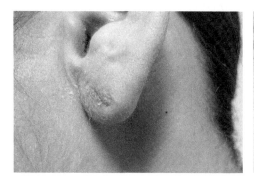
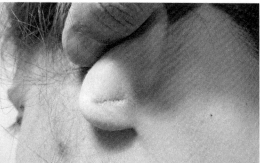

Figure 14.16 Freshened edges approximated using tissue glue (front and back).

- The lesion is excised using a round loop electrode on the blend waveform from its base.
- Hemostasis is achieved with a ball electrode on the electrocoagulation waveform at 4 to 6 power.
- The lesion is allowed to heal with secondary intention.

CAPILLARY HEMANGIOMAS AND PYOGENIC GRANULOMAS

Small vascular lesions over the skin are quite common. A capillary hemangioma occurs without any cause, whereas a pyogenic granuloma usually occurs after some trauma. See Figures 14.17 to 14.20.

- Excision is done under local anesthesia.
- The blend waveform is selected to give a bloodless operative field.
- A round loop electrode is used on power 3 to 6 to excise.
- There could be some oozing after excision.

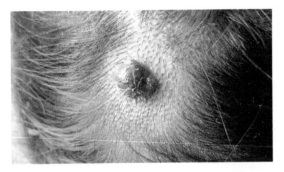

Figure 14.17 Capillary hemangioma on scalp.

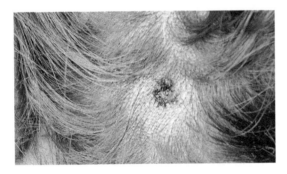

Figure 14.18 Capillary hemangioma excised using blend waveform.

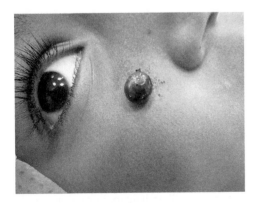

Figure 14.19 Capillary hemangioma on a child.

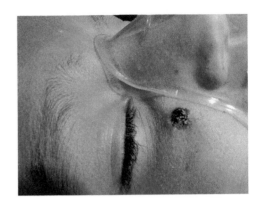

Figure 14.20 Capillary hemangioma on a child is excised in hospital under short general anesthesia.

- The ball electrode is used on the electrocoagulation waveform at 5 to 8 power for hemostasis.
- Blending of edges should be done on a low power of 1 to 2 for all lesions on the face for good cosmetic results.

TRICHOEPITHELIOMAS, NEUROFIBROMAS, AND KERATOACANTHOMAS (CUTANEOUS HORNS)

Trichoepithelioma, neurofibroma, and keratoacanthoma are uncommon. Keratoacanthoma is usually always excised, whereas the other two may be left alone. See Figures 14.21 to 14.24.

- All three lesions have to be excised with a round loop electrode.
- The cut waveform is selected and a power of 3 or 4 is enough for the simple excision.

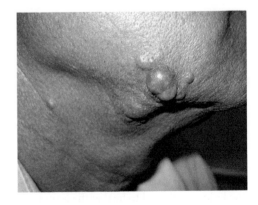

Figure 14.21 Neurofibroma.

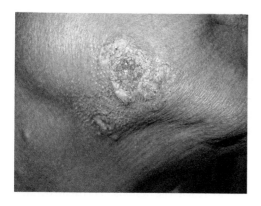

Figure 14.22 Neurofibroma excision.

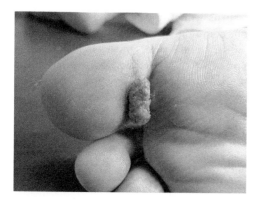

Figure 14.23 Keratoacanthoma.

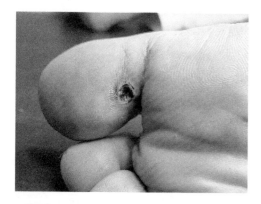

Figure 14.24 Keratoacanthoma excision.

- Lesions of neurofibroma may be deeper and hence can cause some scarring.
- Generally, there will not be much bleeding.
- If required, a ball electrode is used for electro-coagulation on a 5 to 8 power.

- Circumferential blending should be done at low power for good cosmetic result.
- Postoperative wounds are allowed to heal by secondary intention.

FRECKLES

Freckles are small-sized hyperpigmented macules (spots) distributed on sun-exposed areas of the face. They only cause cosmetic disfigurement.

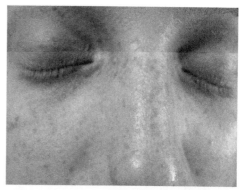

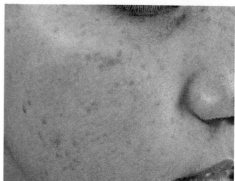

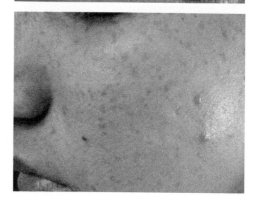

Figure 14.25 Freckles before treatment.

Nowadays, people desire to get rid of them. See Figures 14.25 to 14.26.

- Treatment is done under surface anesthesia.
- Freckles to be treated are marked.
- If the number is very high, it is better to treat in two to three sessions at fortnightly intervals.
- Marked lesions are treated one by one.
- A straight needle electrode is held at 70 to 90 degrees to the skin surface.
- The cut waveform is selected. Power is at 1.
- Very fine strokes are made to the superficial freckles to finely ablate them one by one. Usually, each freckle clears with the perfect fine stroke. Some may remain stuck to the skin surface and fall off after 3 to 4 days.
- Once the freckles have cleared, the face gets a lovely "glow."
- There could be postoperative dyschromia or very shallow scars. Bleaching creams will help alleviate dyschromia. If required,

chemical peels will quickly clear all spots. Shallow scars will also improve fully with chemical peels.

MUCOSAL LESIONS

Mucosal lesions are easily accessible and adjoining mucocutaneous junctions can be very nicely treated with good results. Lesions in nostrils and in the oral cavity (buccal mucosa, tongue) can be treated by bending the electrodes to suit the curvature to reach the lesions. Fortunately, all the electrodes are insulated up to the tip and they are easily bendable at any length of their insulation. Insulation helps in preventing electrical shock and burns while inserting into cavities. Mucosal lesions commonly treated in dermatologic surgery are warts, molluscum, mucoceles, fibromas, and polyps of unknown etiology (for biopsy). These lesions are also present over genital mucosa (especially warts and molluscum). Occasionally, eyelid

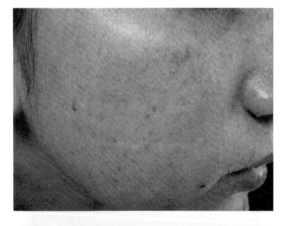
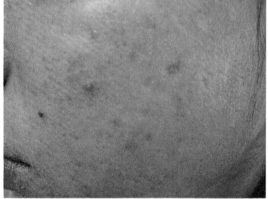
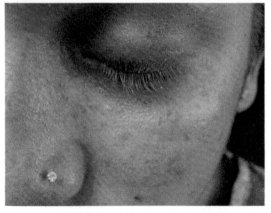
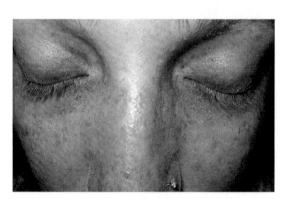

Figure 14.26 After 2 months, the freckles cleared more than 80%.

margins may be involved with warts or molluscum. See Figures 14.27 and 14.28.

- In cases of multiple molluscum or warts, I prefer doing electrodessication with a straight needle electrode or broad needle electrode under surface anesthesia or local anesthesia. All lesions either whiten as mentioned earlier or shrink and darken due to heat. A low power of 1 or 2 is enough. All necrosed lesions will fall off in a week's time. The advantage of this method is there will be no multiple open wounds, which would be painful and likely to get infected.
- Larger warts or molluscum are excised with a round loop electrode or triangular electrode under local anesthesia. Excision is done using the blend waveform.
- Other mentioned lesions that are usually single are excised under local anesthesia.
- Bleeding is less and manageable. Electrocoagulation may occasionally be required. All wounds heal with secondary intention.

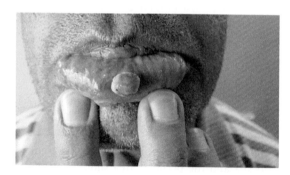

Figure 14.27 Submucous fibroma.

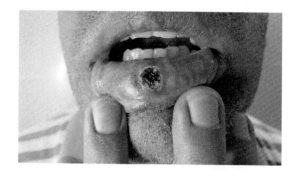

Figure 14.28 The submucous fibroma was excised under local anesthesia.

Let us consider the uncommon applications of RF surgery given in Table 14.2.

HYPERTROPHIC SCARS AND KELOIDS

I prefer to treat both hypertrophic scars and keloids conservatively, especially keloids. But, sometimes due to demand of surgical removal of hypertrophic scars when on exposed areas of the face, neck, arms, and forearms, excision is done. In case of keloids, I refrain from surgical excision unless they are on immobile areas like an earlobe, ear pinna, nose, or forehead. Excision of both is easy, but postoperative care and follow-up is very critical to prevent recurrence. This needs to be emphasized on the patient's mind and only the stable-minded patients with realistic expectations can be selected for excision as a hypertrophic scar can also turn into a keloid after excision if there is a casual approach and improper follow-up. See Figures 14.29 to 14.33.

- Excision is done under local anesthesia.
- The waveform can be cut or blend (choice is individual).
- Power will vary according to the thickness of the lesion.
- Small hypertrophic scars can be easily excised using the shaving technique with a round loop electrode or triangular electrode. These lesions are gradually planed down excising thickened collagen tissue slice by slice to reach a level slightly below the skin surface. Confirm that the thickened collagen tissue is fully excised by visual and tactile sensation.

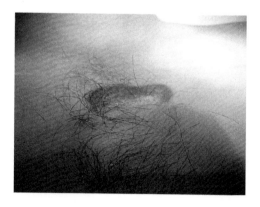

Figure 14.29 Hypertrophic scar.

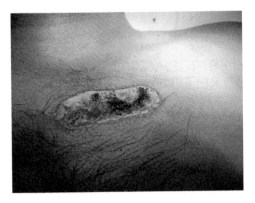

Figure 14.30 The hypertrophic scar was excised under local anesthesia.

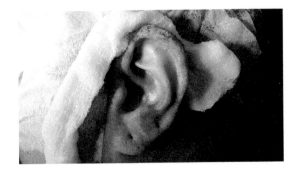

Figure 14.32 Ear keloid immediately after excision.

- Larger hypertrophic scars and keloids are marked first. The border is then incised with the straight needle electrode at the desired edge and the incision is deepened. The edge is held with toothed forceps and the incision is deepened further into the depth of the lesion and along the marked border. Here, care should be taken not to deeply cut the lesion leading to complications or more bleeding. The aim here is to excise most of the thickened collagen tissue but not all. Once the lesion is fully removed, it is viewed under lens and felt for remnants of collagen tissue. The electrode is changed to a round loop or triangular electrode. Using the shaving technique, the remaining collagen tissue is excised until you reach the level just below the skin surface.
- An electrocoagulation waveform along with a ball electrode at power 5 to 10 is used for hemostasis when required.
- I give an injection of triamcinolone 10 mg/ml or 40 mg/ml (choice is individual) immediately

postoperatively, and on the operating table itself in case of a keloid.
- Postoperative wounds are allowed to heal by secondary intention.
- Once the wounds completely heal, patients are advised to apply silicon topical gels twice daily at least for 3 months. Follow-up is done every 2 weeks for 6 months postoperatively and later if required. An injection of Triamcinolone is repeated if required in the healed lesion if there is thickening or itching, and significant inflammation around one month after removal.
- I have used another method for small hypertrophic scars that are round shaped (see page 88).

CONDYLOMA ACUMINATA AND GENITAL LESIONS

Condyloma acuminata affecting male and female genitalia and the perianal area should be treated the same way as given earlier (see "Mucosal Lesions" section). Similarly, other genital lesions are tackled the same way (see "Mucosal Lesions").

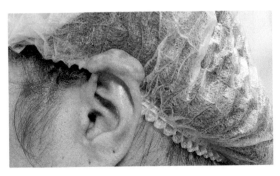

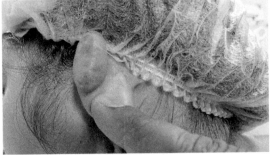

Figure 14.31 Ear keloid.

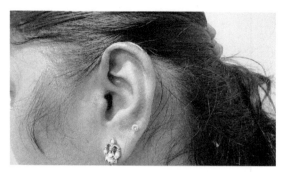

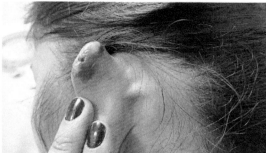

Figure 14.33 Two weeks after excision.

PERIUNGUAL AND SUBUNGUAL LESIONS

There are a number of lesions that are encountered in practice. Most common among them are verrucae or warts. There could be fibroma, hemangioma, hematoma, or recurrent spicules. It is preferable to give ring block anesthesia and use the appropriate electrode for excision. For subungual warts, the nail may have to be cut for a wide excision of these warts. See Figures 14.34 and 14.35.

INGROWN TOENAILS

An ingrown toenail is quite a painful condition. Nowadays many patients approach me for treatment. Incidence seems to have increased due to constant shoe wearing. See Figures 14.36 to 14.39.

- Patient is given a ring block with an injection of lignocaine, and tourniquet is tied proximally to give a bloodless operative field.
- The ingrown toenail is clipped with scissors.

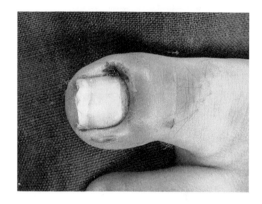

Figure 14.35 The periungual fibroma excised under digital ring block anesthesia.

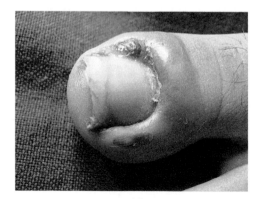

Figure 14.34 Periungual fibroma.

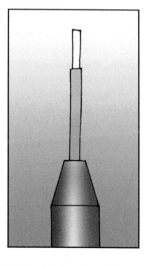

Figure 14.36 Metal side of matrixectomy electrode.

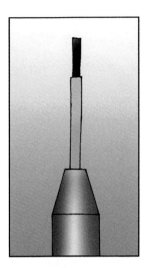

Figure 14.37 Insulated side of matrixectomy electrode.

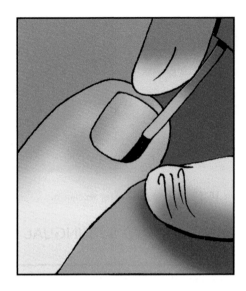

Figure 14.39 Schematic diagram showing how the matrixectomy electrode is inserted while treating an ingrown toenail.

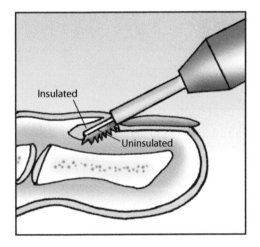

Figure 14.38 Schematic diagram in cross-sectional view showing the insertion of the matrixectomy electrode reaching the germinal epithelium while treating an ingrown toenail.

- A spatula is used to separate the proximal nail fold from the underlying nail plate.
- Similarly, the nail plate is separated from the nail bed on that side immediately.
- The cut nail plate is gripped with hemostat forceps and firmly pulled out. Confirm that no portion is left behind.
- Curette is scraped on the nail bed to remove granulations.

- A nail matrixectomy electrode has one side insulated and the other bare (noninsulated). This electrode is inserted inside keeping its metal (noninsulated side) touching the germinal epithelium and the insulated side upward against the eponychium (thus prevents damage to eponychium).
- The waveform of electrocoagulation is selected and a power of 5 or 6 is set. The current is applied for 3 to 5 seconds holding the electrode slightly away for best results. The electrode is gradually removed.
- This destroys the germinal epithelium. This step is most critical for successful results. If done improperly, there is recurrence.
- Pressure dressing is done and removed after 2 days. Afterwards the dressings are changed on every alternate day until healing is complete.
- Follow-up is done every 2 weeks for a minimum of 3 months.

RHINOPHYMA

Rhinophyma[1] is a nasal disfigurement that causes great cosmetic distress to the patient. Conservative treatment never works here. The overgrown tissue causing the large, red, bumpy nose should be planed down to reshape the nose to relieve the patient from cosmetic disfigurement. See Figures 14.40 to 14.42.

- Local anesthesia is injected at various points around the nose as shown in Figure 14.41.
- Blend waveform and round loop electrode are selected.

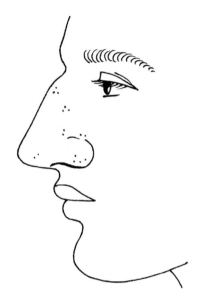

Figure 14.42 Two to three months after treatment (schematic drawing).

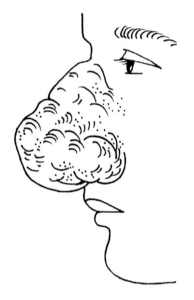

Figure 14.40 Rhinophyma (schematic drawing).

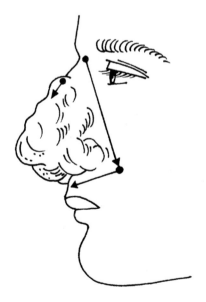

Figure 14.41 How local anesthesia is given around the nose.

- A power of 3 to 6 should be sufficient to resect the overgrown or hypertrophic nasal tissue.
- The shave technique is used for excision. The excess sebaceous tissue is excised slice after slice using paintbrush-like strokes to reshape the nose. It is an artist like job where you are literally restoring the patient's nose back to a normal shape.
- I always take care to study the patient's shape of nose beforehand from his or her earlier photos. After a few down strokes, I always study the improvement from all angles on the operating table. One has to make a tangential observation from all sides.
- Nasal contour and symmetry should be reestablished as far as possible, but overzealous cutting must be avoided.
- Bleeding is hardly a problem while operating.
- The postoperative wound is allowed to heal by secondary intention.
- Wound healing may require 3 to 4 weeks.

FACIAL GRAY HAIR

Radiofrequency waves being colorblind are best to deal with gray hair hirsutism. Gray facial hair becomes a problem in middle and old age. Lasers being wavelength specific are best for black hair.

- Very thin wire electrodes (hair removing electrodes) are available in two to three sizes.
- These electrodes are specially manufactured to protect the adjoining epidermis and dermis while inserting and passing RF waves to hair roots by Teflon insulation right up to the tip. Only the tip is exposed.
- The process of treating each gray hair is a bit tedious and laborious, but the results are as good as lasers.
- The electrode is selected depending upon the thickness of facial gray hair.
- The waveform is electrocoagulation.
- Power is 1.
- Working under magnifying lens, the electrode is pushed along the hair shaft inside in the direction of the hair to reach the hair root. There is a slight resistance when one reaches the hair root. Stopping then, activate the foot pedal for just a second or two. This discharges radio waves to the root and there will be a small sound of spark, which indicates the hair root is coagulated (or burnt). Remove the electrode and continue this process for other gray hairs (Figure 14.43).
- Gradually pull out the hair with tweezers.
- Occasionally a drop of blood may ooze out after pulling out the hair; just wipe with normal saline.

- Pain is very mild and does not require topical anesthesia.
- Results are very good; there is no scarring.

CHRONIC LICHENIFIED ECZEMA, PRURIGO NODULARIS, HYPERTROPHIC LICHEN PLANUS, AND PAPULAR OR NODULAR LESION OF UNKNOWN ETIOLOGY

These lesions are some of the most distressing and recalcitrant lesions that are resistant to a medical line of treatment. They can be intensely pruritic. Intralesional injections of triamcinolone or hydrocortisone are effective but may not be able to prevent recurrence, and repeated injections may cause depigmentation. Surgical excision using radiofrequency technique is a very good option in selected cases. The major obstacle or disadvantage in doing so is that these lesions being almost always on the legs and ankles, postoperative wounds cause major discomfort and pain. This may restrict the patient's activity until wound healing occurs. I have treated a few dozen cases of these on legs and ankles after proper planning. If lesions are bilateral, the lesions on one foot or ankle are tackled first and then the other foot or ankle after a month to allow for patient's movements. The results are usually gratifying. Patients should be followed up every 2 weeks for 2 months and later once a month for 3 to

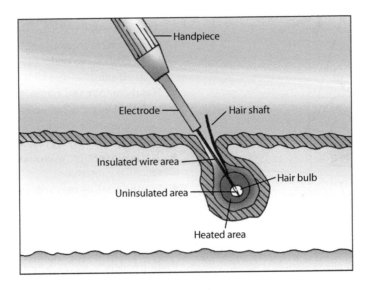

Figure 14.43 Gray hair epilation technique (schematic drawing).

4 months. Recurrence is unlikely when follow-up is good. See Figures 14.44 to 14.54.

- Injection of lignocaine 2% with adrenaline is given underneath the selected lesions.
- Lesions are excised fully using the cut or blend waveform at 3 to 8 power depending upon the thickness of the lesions. A triangular or round loop electrode is best.

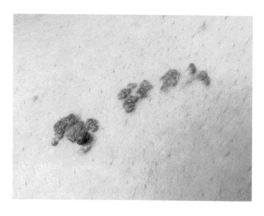

Figure 14.46 Epidermal nevus on chest area.

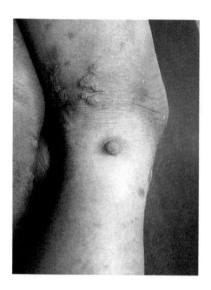

Figure 14.44 Prurigo nodularis.

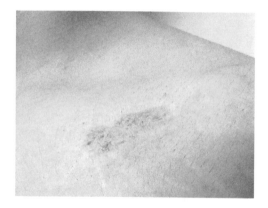

Figure 14.47 Epidermal nevus on chest area excised.

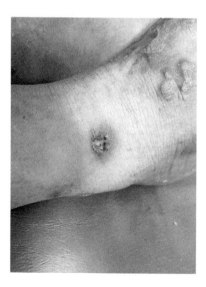

Figure 14.45 Prurigo nodularis lesion completely excised.

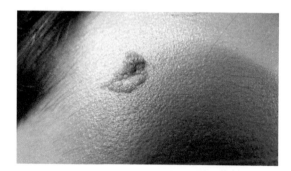

Figure 14.48 Epidermal nevus on forehead.

- When the blend waveform is used, there is no bleeding. In case of bleeding, hemostasis is achieved with the ball electrode at 5 or 6 power.
- Postoperative wounds heal well with secondary intention.
- Dressing may be required daily until the wound heals.

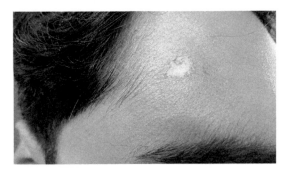

Figure 14.49 Epidermal nevus on forehead excised.

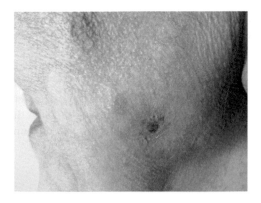

Figure 14.52 Two weeks after cutaneous horn excision.

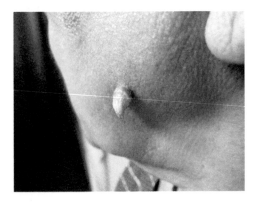

Figure 14.50 Cutaneous horn.

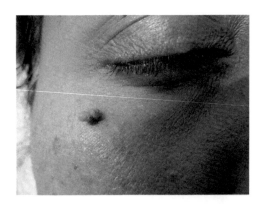

Figure 14.53 Tuberculous verrucosa cutis.

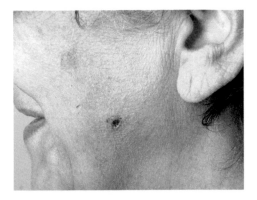

Figure 14.51 The cutaneous horn was excised under local anesthesia.

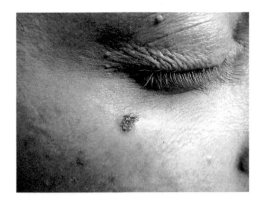

Figure 14.54 Tuberculous verrucosa cutis finely excised.

- Chances of sepsis are quite high since postoperative wound healing is commonly delayed due to movements that slow the rate of granulation tissue formation.
- Recurrence will not occur so easily unless the wounds take a long time to heal or there is sepsis, which leads to hypertrophy of scars.

- In case of such a problem, such scars are treated aggressively with potent topical steroids to reduce hypertrophy.
- Except for the aforementioned problem, postoperative scars are otherwise thin and acceptable. Sometimes there could be atrophic scars.

Papular and nodular lesions of unknown etiology are sent for biopsy using RF excisional biopsy technique (refer to Chapter 16).

TELANGIECTASIA

Telangiectasia, or thread veins or spider nevus, can be very effectively treated using radiofrequency surgery. The technique is very simple and quick to perform. Facial telangiectasia (Figure 14.55) respond better than thread veins on thighs or legs.

- Surface anesthesia is optional because pain during the procedure is momentary and very much bearable.
- Electrocoagulation waveform is selected.
- A special telangiectasia electrode is available with Teflon insulation up to the tip. It looks similar to that which is used for gray hair removal.
- Power used is 1.
- The electrode can be bent to the angle required to facilitate procedure.
- Under magnifying lens, the veins to be treated are selected and the foot pedal is depressed continuously while the electrode is finely touched upon the length of veins at small intervals of 2 to 3 mm just for a second one after another.
- Mild bleeding may occur occasionally; stops with pressure.
- Usually, the treated veins become blanched and may later disappear completely within a week. Sometimes, more than one session is required.
- There is no scab formation. Intraoperative pain is bearable, and there is no postoperative pain.
- Results are excellent.

BASAL CELL CARCINOMA

Clinically obvious basal cell carcinoma lesions on the face of small size are selected for excision biopsy. I prefer to avoid treating lesions very close to the eyes. For lesions on the nose, I prefer to do an incisional biopsy to confirm diagnosis and not do a full excision because of the critical shape of the nose, which can be perfectly restored by plastic or cosmetic surgeons after wide local excision. See Figures 14.56 and 14.57.

- Lesions are excised under local anesthesia.
- The blend waveform is preferred.

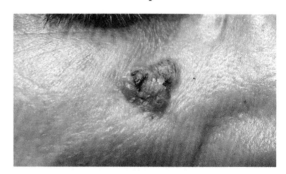

Figure 14.56 Basal cell carcinoma.

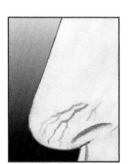
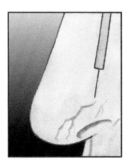
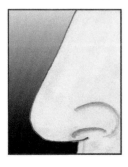

Figure 14.55 Facial telangiectasia treatment (schematic drawing).

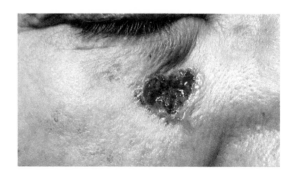

Figure 14.57 Basal cell carcinoma (excision biopsy).

- When doing incisional biopsy, I prefer doing it using the cut waveform to best preserve tissue architecture.
- Round loop electrode is selected.
- Before excising, I plan to make the first cut to remove the maximum amount of lesion from the depth in one stroke.
- Power should be at least 5 or 6 for the blend waveform and 3 or 4 for the cut waveform.
- The round loop electrode is just pushed without pressure smoothly right from the depth of the lesion to remove as large a piece as possible.
- This piece is transferred to a formol saline bottle to be sent to histopathology.
- The rest of the lesion is then fully removed using multiple soft strokes cutting piece by piece.

- In spite of the blend waveform, some capillary bleeding is expected.
- Hemostasis is achieved with the ball electrode in the electrocoagulation waveform.
- Dressing and postoperative care as usual.
- Once the histopathology report gives confirmation of basal cell carcinoma, the patient will have to be referred to an oncosurgeon for further action.

REFERENCE

1. Clarke DP, Hanker CW. Electrosurgical treatment of rhinophyma. *J Am Acid Dermatol* 1990; 22:831–837.

15

Gems and jewels of radiofrequency surgery

Radiofrequency surgery is a marvelous technique. One can make effective use of all of its parts and functions to develop newer and novel applications. One can use the various waveforms for different indications, change electrodes to suit applications, bend electrodes to reach inside cavities or avoid adjacent tissue damage, use power from a minimum of 0.5–1 to 100 on a digital unit, perform small-hole surgeries, do epilation, do biopsies, and nowadays with flat or large dome-shaped electrodes do skin tightening in cosmetic dermatology.

While using the radiofrequency technique in practice I noticed that when I used it on a low power of 1 or 2 on the cut waveform and apply the round loop electrode finely at the margins of a depressed scar, I could literally shape the uneven skin surface of the scar at its edge to look better. Similarly, when I keep the thin wire electrode or straight needle electrode inside the bulk of the lesion (e.g., sebaceous cyst, neurofibroma, keloid) to be excised, kept the power above 4, and pressed the foot pedal for a few seconds, the concerned tissue would shrink or contract and flatten quickly to more than half of its original size. These two observations were amazing. I noticed this while working and experimenting in my early days of using radiofrequency surgery way back in 2000–2001.

This is how I started experimenting on deep, punched out scars of acne and trauma on the face. The ablative Er:YAG laser had just entered the aesthetic market to compete with the already present ablative CO_2 laser. These were being used for acne scars then and dermatologists were learning these new aesthetic applications. Both lasers worked on the principle of photothermal vaporization.

While working on depressed or atrophic scars, I noticed that these scars had uneven or punched out edges that cast a shadow giving an ugly and unsightly appearance on the face. This shadowing effect was due to light physics that failed to reach the angulated portion of the edges of scars in the same intensity as the adjacent plane skin and the floor of the scars. The shadowing effect depends upon the angle from which the light falls on the scar. Light falling from the front, that is, perpendicular to the skin surface where the scar is, causes less shadowing effect compared to when falling from one of the sides or when there is uneven light in the same room or when it is twilight or when one is viewing the same scar in a room under artificial tube lights or LED lights. Hence, the most important defect that needed correction was the sloping or punched out or uneven scar edges. If these could be improved or resurfaced to alleviate their slope, angle, and unevenness, then much was expected to improve the shape of scars to allow more light inside leading to an improved appearance. This was a matter of *artistic use of the radiofrequency method* to cause this resurfacing.

This idea of artistic use of RF method to significantly alleviate the shadowing effect was boosted by understanding the working of microdermabrasion. The microdermabrasion technique causes buffing of the skin surface to polish the skin surface, but the handpiece, which either delivers crystals or has diamond fraises when it touches the skin surface, pulls up the skin inside the small hole by the vacuum developed in the machine. When working with the microdermabrasion technique for some acne scars giving some overlap passes at the scar borders, I observed that some resurfacing of these borders was occurring to lessen the shadowing effect, and the scars appeared somewhat improved in three to four treatments. This I guess was not just due to the buffing effect but also to the pulling of uneven scar skin inside the probe by the vacuum generated and mechanically finely abrading the skin at edges to soften sharp edges. This simple technique allowed more light inside the scar to give the virtual effect of improvement without the scar floor getting uplifted.

I experimented further with this idea on a few more patients with deep scars on the face and elsewhere. I tried using a low power and round loop electrode on scar edges stretching the skin between two fingers of the inactive hand under local anesthesia. This led to widening of the scar dimensions, though the edges looked smoother than before and the shadowing effect did lessen.

After more experimentation, I finally came to the conclusion that if I lifted the selected deep scar between the index finger and thumb of the inactive hand and worked on the scar edges to level and soften the sharpness of edges or borders, I could find the virtual scar improvement effect much better without widening of the scar dimensions.

I realized that to improve selected deep and punched out scars I should be able to lift the scar between two fingers to a critical height so that the scar floor is also lifted in the pinch and looks flat or slightly convex. Only if I could hold this position, then I could go further to soften the edges.

Softening of sharp edges was done with a round loop electrode using the cut waveform and power set at 3 or 4. This was bloodless. This was a fine cutting or ablation and not abrasion. The ablation was continued on the whole circumference of the scar. The point to note here is that the convexity of the adjacent normal skin made cutting edges and leveling much easier than when there was concavity due to stretching of skin.

I would like to compare this observation with a saucer design for better understanding. I would compare stretching of a scar to a regular saucer design where the cutting with electrode would likely give a widening effect (Figure 15.1). Whereas, I would compare lifting of a scar to an inverted saucer design (Figure 15.2), where the cutting would lead to better softening of sharp edges and better blending with adjacent skin. This edge ablation is done until the sharp edge is made blunt and scar

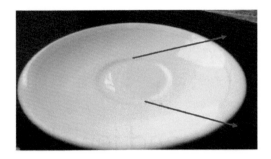

Figure 15.1 Saucer compared to depressed punched out scar on face. Arrows point in direction of strokes used to blunt sharp edges, but stretching scar and using this technique widens the scar.

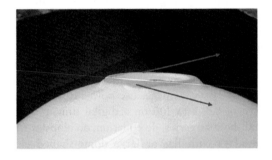

Figure 15.2 Saucer upside down indicates the lifted up scar and arrows point in direction of strokes used to blunt sharp edges. This does not widen the scar and gives a much better resurfacing effect.

floor level (plane) almost matches with the adjacent skin level (plane).

To further improve upon this technique, I experimented on two more aspects, namely, the scar floor and adjacent skin.

After experimenting on different depressed and atrophic facial scars with proper photo documentation, I finally developed my own method of scar resurfacing with radiofrequency. I helped improve a number of such facial scars of different varieties including chicken pox scars, acne scars (selected), and posttraumatic scars. I presented my original work at many national and international conferences from 2002, including the National Dermatology Conference conducted by the Indian Association of Dermatologists, Venereologists and Leprologists at Cochin in India and the 20th World Congress of Dermatology in Paris.

I soon developed a similar resurfacing method for hypertrophic scars and keloids, where I stretched the scar before resurfacing.

RADIOFREQUENCY RESURFACING TECHNIQUE FOR DEPRESSED FACIAL SCARS

Radiofrequency resurfacing for depressed facial scars[1] needs proper learning and practice to get good results. This technique is a maneuver that is implemented in three steps. It is performed under local anesthesia of an injection of lignocaine 2% with adrenaline. Scars need to be selected for best results. I recommend this technique for resurfacing the deep and punched out facial scars of acne, trauma, and chicken pox.

Selection criteria:
* Deep scars of a minimum 4–5 mm and not more than 1.5 cm width.
* Depth of scars should be more than 1 mm.

Stepwise procedure

* Primary preparations are made as usual.
* Local anesthesia is given under and around scar.
* The scar is marked with a marker pen.
* Electrodes used for this can be any of the following: surgical round blade or flat round Surgipen (see Chapter 10, Figure 10.10) preferably. A round loop electrode can be used if the other electrodes are not available.
* A cut waveform is used.

STEP 1: SCAR EDGE ABLATION FOR LEVELING

* See Figures 15.3.
* Power is set to 3 or 4.
* The scar is lifted between the index finger and thumb of the inactive hand to a critical height as described earlier.
* The scar edges are ablated all around holding the electrode at 75 to 90 degrees to the skin surface plane.
* The end point will be close matching of levels of scar floor and adjacent skin.
* The operative field remains bloodless.

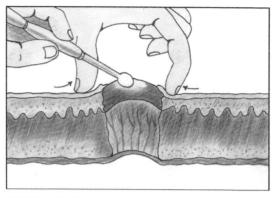

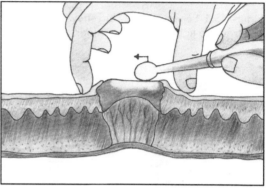

Figure 15.3 Schematic drawing showing angle of holding Surgipen to blunt edges.

STEP 2: SCAR FLOOR ABLATION FOR COLLAGEN REMODELING TO IMPROVE DEPTH

* See Figure 15.4.
* Scar lifting is continued as above and the scar floor is finely ablated in a single pass.
* Power remains at 3 or 4.
* There is no bleeding.

STEP 3: CIRCUMFERENTIAL BLENDING FOR HOMOGENOUS BLENDING WITH ADJACENT SKIN

* See Figure 15.5.
* Scar lifting is continued as above.
* Power is kept at 1 or 2. Here, there is no ablation.
* The electrode is very lightly and finely stroked over the ablated edge first (circumferential blending) and later from the ablated edges toward the adjacent normal skin in the centrifugal direction (centrifugal blending).

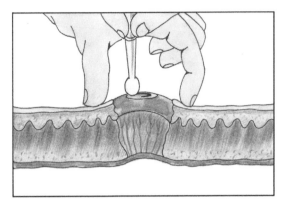

Figure 15.4 Schematic drawing showing angle of electrode to lightly ablate scar floor.

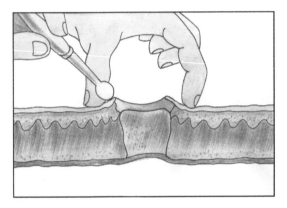

Figure 15.5 Schematic drawing showing angle of electrode while working from edge of scar to adjoining normal.

- Here, the aim is not to cut or ablate, but to shape or sculpt the adjacent normal skin at the edges to lessen demarcation of the scar to make it diffuse.
- While performing this step, the border is visibly reshaped to nicely blend into the scar edge.

The resurfaced scars are allowed to heal by secondary intention. Wounds are kept open. Antibiotic ointment is applied and standard postoperative care is taken.

The wounds heal within 8 to 10 days. Postoperative dyschromia is possible (hyperpigmentation on Fitzpatrick skin types 3 to 5 and erythema on skin types 1 and 2). This generally develops approximately 3 to 4 weeks after the procedure. Hyperpigmentation finally clears with bleaching creams within 1 to 2 months. There will be no residual pigment.

Final results are best achieved by the end of 2 months (Figures 15.6 to 15.8).

Scar improvement is expected to be seen in all cases. Virtual improvement in the depth of the scar is seen in up to 50% to 60% in most of the treated scars. Scar edges soften remarkably, reducing the shadowing effect significantly. This improvement is achieved in a single maneuver, which is a great advantage.

Results are best over cheeks. It is difficult to achieve similar results over the forehead and nose because of the difficulty in lifting up the scar.

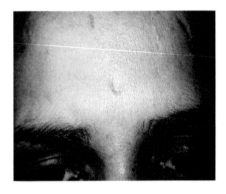

Figure 15.6 Small depressed scar on central forehead of many years duration.

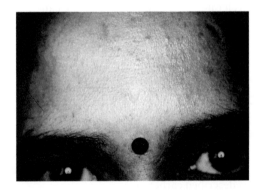

Figure 15.7 Excellent resurfacing effect (more than 80% improvement in scar depth) in one session.

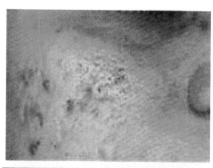
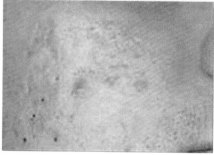

Figure 15.8 Excellent resurfacing effect observed (selective resurfacing of deeper scars was done).

RADIOFREQUENCY RESURFACING TECHNIQUE FOR HYPERTROPHIC SCARS ON FACE

Patients having hypertrophic scars and keloids often approach for treatment. I do only very selective excision of keloids, whereas I excise all hypertrophic scars. Facial hypertrophic scars can be excised very easily and quickly.

- Primary preparations are done as usual.
- Local anesthesia of lignocaine 2% with adrenaline is given underneath the lesion.
- A cut or blend is used at a power of 3 to 6.
- A round loop electrode is best. For larger scars, a straight needle electrode is better to first excise the larger portion of scar holding it with tooth forceps.
- Skin around the hypertrophic scar is stretched before excision.
- If a straight needle electrode is used, the lesion's borders are first marked with the electrode itself. Cutting is started at one end and

gradually the whole scar is excised holding it with toothed forceps.
- Bleeding is very little.
- Later, a round loop electrode is inserted in the handpiece and the remaining portion of the scar is excised piece by piece until all of the thickened scar tissue is fully removed.
- The postoperative wound is allowed to heal by secondary intention.
- The wound usually heals in 2 weeks.
- Good follow-up is a must to prevent it from recurrence. Topical silicone gels must be advised for regular application on a twice daily basis for a long duration of at least 3 to 6 months.
- In case of any early signs of recurrence, I would recommend use of an injection of triamcinolone intralesionally.

RADIOVAPORIZATION AND ITS APPLICATIONS

In earlier chapters when I mentioned the working of the radiofrequency technique, I had said that tissue resistance to passage of radio waves creates heat. This heat is due to extreme intracellular water molecular vibrations. This heat finally leads to bursting of cells and eventually cutting or necrosis of tissues concerned. The same principle when applied in a different manner causes an interesting phenomenon of tissue vaporization leading to a shrinking or debulking effect.

I mentioned earlier the application of electrodessication in which the tissue dehydrates and shrinks to become necrosed. Here, the electrode is applied externally, which creates tissue vaporization leading to dehydration.

The same application if done on a cut waveform at a higher power of more than 3 or 4 using a straight needle electrode inserted inside a cyst or small hypertrophic scar or keloid or a submucous cyst or a neurofibroma will vaporize the soft tissues inside the lesions causing it to shrink more than half its size within a few seconds. This facilitates excision of such lesions. Dr. Chiarello[2] used this technique for many lesions, such as rhinophyma, and observed that it could help sculpting tissues. He used a "hockey stick electrode" and much higher power.

I have been using straight needle and thin wire electrodes for certain cysts like sebaceous and submucous as well as for small hypertrophic scars and keloids. In cysts, it causes collapse of the cyst wall due to vaporization of its contents, whereas in scars it causes vaporization and denaturation of its collagen and ground substance leading to remarkable shrinkage of the same. This makes excision easy. Sometimes in small sebaceous cysts this much may be enough, as extracting the cyst wall and excising it is avoided and there is no recurrence. However, there is the possibility of a small depressed scar if the cyst is large. All these procedures are done under local anesthesia.

REFERENCES

1. Deshpande B. Single step maneuver of radiofrequency resurfacing for selected deep and punched out scars on face. In: F056: Late-Breaking Research: Surgical and Cosmetic; 73rd American Academy of Dermatology, 2015.
2. Chiarello SE. Radiovaporization: Radiofrequency cutting current to vaporize and sculpt skin lesions. *Dermatol Surg* 2003; 29:755–758.

16

Biopsy using radiofrequency surgery

A skin biopsy should not only be performed when one suspects malignancy, but as a routine for many of the common skin lesions surgically removed in practice. Simultaneously, a biopsy is done many times to diagnose a skin disease when eluding diagnosis or when the given treatment fails to give expected results.

A skin biopsy has been commonly done using a scalpel or curette or punches of various sizes. As noted earlier, techniques of electrocautery, cryotherapy, and lasers are not suitable for biopsy, though cryotherapy may be used in some cases.

Radiofrequency surgery serves as a good option for doing a skin biopsy. Since the time I started this technique, I noticed that lesions removed had the skin structure very nicely preserved, as the cut is very fine. After observing this, I thought of using this for excision biopsy, which succeeded. The histopathology report remarked that the tissue architecture was well preserved except for some thermal changes at margins.

It has been proved in various scientific studies that radiofrequency surgery has one of the thinnest cuts (10–20 microns).[1,2]

Gradually, as I developed more experience using radiofrequency surgery in practice, I stopped using punch for biopsy. Using punch for biopsy only became cumbersome, so I omitted it from practice.

Using radiofrequency surgery I could use the same tool for treatment as well as diagnosis. I have since then used it for all cases of excisional and incisional biopsies. The results have been very satisfactory.

I started with simple cases of corns and warts. Once I was convinced with all the reports, I started expanding this application to moles and skin tags. Over the next 1 to 2 years, I used it for diagnosing

clinical dermatologic conditions like psoriasis and lichen planus with very satisfactory results.

Using it for elevated dermatologic conditions was easier. I then decided to use it on flat lesions like unexplained hypopigmented or hyperpigmented macules and was convinced that I could reach the depth of the lower dermis while excising the biopsy piece from such macules in a single perfect stroke.

The next step was to use it to diagnose cases of leprosy, which is very common in India. This worked out very well. Since then, I have been using it for all cases of doubtful and frank leprosy with very good results. It was possible to get the proper classification of leprosy as well as tuberculoid or lepromatous and its subtypes.

The next step was to try it on blistering or vesiculobullous disorders. This was a challenging task, as to take biopsy for these disorders required making a cut deep enough to excise the recent vesicle in toto from its base and taking it without bursting. Conditions like pemphigus vulgaris, which have very superficial and flaccid bullae, was tough. Here and in macular lesions, the advantage was of using a larger size round loop electrode to reach beyond the base of the bullae into adjacent skin and to reach deeper dermis.

Finally, I decided to use it to diagnose cases of malignancy and basal cell carcinoma. Here, the cut needs to be sufficiently deep and wide as well to involve adjacent normal skin.

Vascular lesions like capillary hemangiomas and pyogenic granulomas were effectively excised for biopsy as well.

This is how radiofrequency surgery was incorporated in my practice as a diagnostic tool. I have always used the cut or fully filtered waveform at a power of 3 to 6. I prefer the round loop, straight needle, or thin wire electrodes, though one can always use the electrode of their choice (except for the broad needle electrode).

I have provided clinical photographs of lesions taken for biopsy and a range of histopathology photomicrographs for your perusal (Figures 16.1 to 16.14).

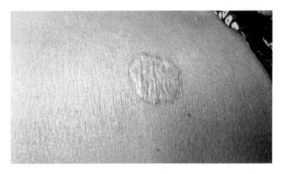

Figure 16.1 Hypoaesthetic plaque of tuberculoid leprosy.

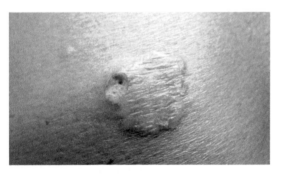

Figure 16.2 Incisional biopsy taken from the edge of the plaque including normal skin.

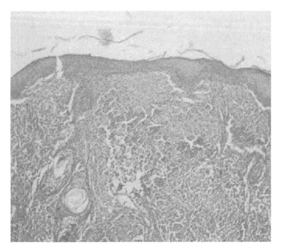

Figure 16.3 Tuberculoid leprosy.

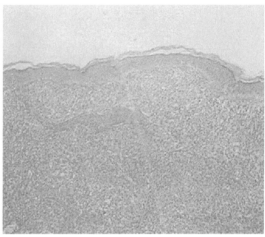

Figure 16.4 Borderline lepromatous leprosy.

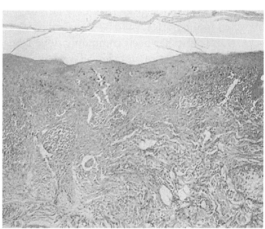

Figure 16.5 Lichen planus.

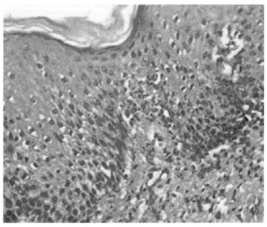

Figure 16.6 Linear IgA bullous disease.

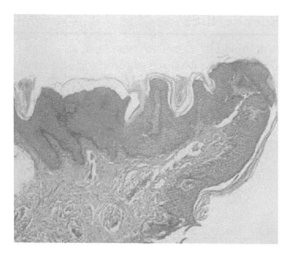

Figure 16.7 Epidermal nevus.

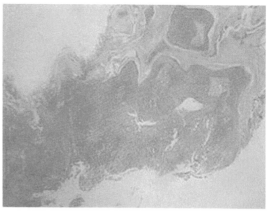

Figure 16.10 Seborrheic keratosis.

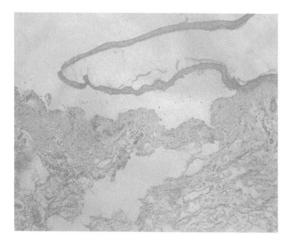

Figure 16.8 Bullous pemphigoid.

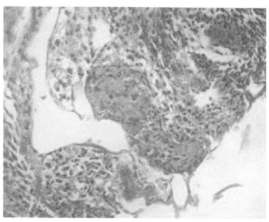

Figure 16.11 Cutaneous tuberculosis.

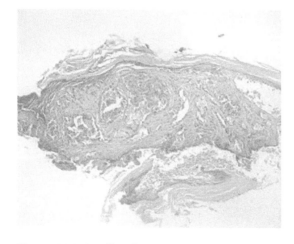

Figure 16.9 Capillary hemangioma.

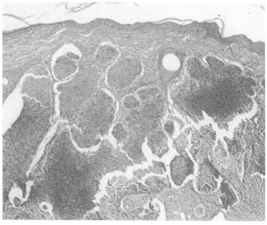

Figure 16.12 Basal cell carcinoma.

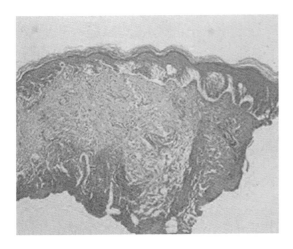

Figure 16.13 Lichen planopilaris.

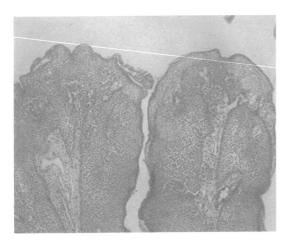

Figure 16.14 Condyloma acuminata.

REFERENCES

1. Turner RJ, Cohen RA, Viet RL et al. Analysis of margins of cone biopsy specimens obtained with "cold knife," CO2 and Nd:YAG lasers and a radiofrequency surgical unit. *J Reproductive Med* 1992; 37:607–610.
2. Maness WL, Roeber FW, Clarke RE et al. Histological evaluation of electrosurgery with varying frequency and waveform. *J Prosthetic Dent* 1978; 40:304–308.

17

Postoperative recovery and care

Postoperative recovery is same as that for any other skin surgery as far as wound healing by secondary intention is concerned. All postoperative wounds on the face generally take a maximum of 1 week to heal, whereas that on other areas take at least 3 or 4 days more. Wounds on the back and feet take the longest time (at least 2 weeks) to heal. Wounds on the scalp also heal within 1 week. Larger and deeper wounds take a longer time to heal.

All patients are very impatient. They expect to recover very fast. Many do not understand the importance of wound care and follow-up. Many patients think that once the surgical procedure is complete, everything is done and the rest of the things will follow automatically. Hence, I feel it is our responsibility to explain and emphasize upon their minds that surgery is only the first half of the process. If patients wish to recover fast and best, they should understand the importance of proper postoperative wound care. Simultaneously, when patients expect a good cosmetic result, it is equally important for them to understand that wound healing until new skin formation (reepithelialization) is just 1 to 2 weeks, whereas the new scar formation process (collagen remodeling stage) lasts for 45 to 60 days depending upon the area of the body. If postoperative advice is not properly followed, the possibility of ugly scarring increases. Hence, I always incorporate this information about postoperative care and follow-up in all my informed consent forms, which I always explain to my patients in detail beforehand. I have worried about my illiterate and poor patients not following instructions and thus getting into trouble, but this has happened very occasionally with them, because even if they are unable to read they listen to verbal advice very carefully and follow meticulously. In contrast, some of the well-off, aristocratic, well-read, well-informed patients do not follow postoperative advice and care properly, and may land into trouble with scarring.

GENERAL POSTOPERATIVE CARE (EXCISION WOUNDS)

- Wound dressing is done immediately postoperatively.
- Dressing should be done daily except for some conditions (e.g., ingrown toenail surgery).
- Oral antibiotic (choice can vary), such as Cefixime, Cefpodoxime, Cefuroxime Axetil, Ofloxacin, Levofloxacin, Ciprofloxacin, Azithromycin, or Roxithromycin, is given for 5 to 10 days.
- Pain-relieving medicines nonsteroidal anti-inflammatory drugs (NSAIDs) are usually not required much except for cases of corns, calluses, palmar or plantar warts, keloids, hypertrophic scars, basal cell carcinoma, bigger or multiple lesions, and mucosal lesions.
- A head bath should be avoided for at least one week for all scalp lesions.
- Wounds on the feet or soles require extra precautions from wetting and bathing as well as dust.
- All facial wounds should be covered with the smallest of dressings, because the patient may be embarrassed by big dressing and can be left open once the wound dries.
- Topical antibiotic of fusidic acid or mupirocin or nadifloxacin is advised for dressing.
- Superficial abrasions following facial scar resurfacing need not be dressed. Application of one of the topical antibiotics listed above is enough.
- Soap should be avoided until wound healing is complete. Nonsoapy washes, like a combination of cetyl and steryl alcohol, is preferred to prevent irritation.

GENERAL POSTOPERATIVE CARE (DESICCATION WOUNDS)

- These lesions may or may not be fully removed immediately after treatment. There is no dressing, even though some of the lesions are wiped off lightly after treatment, the wounds are very small and superficial. I apply postprocedure soothing gels immediately after treatment.
- Overall, all desiccated lesions are left alone to fall off automatically. This should be stressed to patients, as they always want to get rid of the lesions hastily and hence may play with the scabs or excoriate them. Patients should know that any premature exfoliation of postoperative scabs may cause secondary infection and eventually scarring.
- I prefer giving a short course of oral steroids like Deflazacort 6 mg twice daily or Methylprednisolone 4 mg tablet twice daily for 3 days to immediately control postoperative erythema and inflammation. This helps in quickly reducing postoperative discomfort and preventing postinflammatory hyperpigmentation later.
- All patients should try to postpone important events like meetings, interviews, and social programs for a week after treatment on the face or neck, as all lesions will not have fallen off until then.
- Topical antibiotic fucidic acid or mupirocin or nadifloxacin is advised to be applied twice daily until all scabs fall off.
- Oral antibiotics mentioned earlier should be given for a week when many lesions have been treated or if the patient is diabetic.
- Pain-relieving medicines are generally not required.

AFTERCARE

All wounds once healed do require aftercare. I recommend strict aftercare for lesions on the face, neck, upper limbs, and other exposed areas for the significance of wound cosmesis. Even postoperative dyschromia can cause worry in these areas. This aftercare is for prevention of complications and enhancing the quality of the final result.

The following aftercare is recommended:

- All treated areas must be protected from sunlight with the help of a good quality sunscreen (SPF >40). Patients working out in sunlight for long hours should reapply sunscreen every 2 hours.
- A nonsoapy cleansing lotion may be continued or a gentle syndet-based soap should be used.
- If any hyperpigmentation is noticed on treated areas during the follow-up visit, immediate use of good quality bleaching creams should be recommended to clear it.
- Loose clothing and undergarments should be recommended in cases of groin, thigh, and buttock lesions.
- For plantar lesions, excess standing and walking should be avoided for at least 3 months postoperatively to prevent recurrence. A softening agent or emollient should be applied on healed wounds postoperatively to prevent hardening of tissues. Here, barefoot walking should be avoided.
- If there appears to be a possibility of scarring, immediate measures to alleviate scar formation must be taken.

18

Tips and tricks to minimize complications

Dermatologic surgery is fortunate not to have systemic complications as in other surgical specialties. That should not be an excuse for being casual in approach as any dermatologic surgery done without planning, with improper technique or equipment, or by inexperienced clinicians have potential to cause permanent complications on the skin. Though complications of scarring are far less with radiofrequency surgery does not mean one is safe.

COMPLICATIONS DUE TO ANESTHETICS

Before I discuss the postsurgical complications, I would like to caution about problems that may occur due to local anesthetic. Both surface and local injectable anesthesia can cause complications of allergy. Surface anesthesia using cream of lidocaine and prilocaine can occasionally cause itching, burning, or swelling on application. Though this is very rare, if noticed one must wipe it off immediately and clean the area thoroughly with nonsoapy cleanser. In that case the procedure may have to be postponed if the inflammation or rash is significant. Sometimes, a patient does not report mild symptoms before the procedure but reports it later when we will notice more-than-expected inflammation on the operated sites. This may lead to postinflammatory dyschromia. I have never seen vesicular eruption to surface anesthesia. The allergic manifestations can be easily noticed on eyelids than other areas when treating periocular lesions of milia, syringoma, and molluscum. I have experienced only nine cases of allergy to surface

anesthesia in my use over 12 years. Injectable local anesthesia of lignocaine 2% with or without adrenaline may cause problems from vasovagal shock to frank anaphylaxis. Hence, a presurgical test dose is a must. Informing patients and relatives about such complications when the test dose is given is mandatory for immediate reporting.

COMPLICATIONS DUE TO EQUIPMENT, ELECTRICAL INAPPROPRIATENESS, AND ELECTRODE PROBLEMS

Though the complications are uncommon, one should be aware of the following:

- Equipment may stop working unexpectedly while doing surgery. This happens very rarely, and surgery will have to be performed using other equipment (which can never match the same features) and hence results are affected. I have had this experience once while working with my equipment when in between surgery of a mole I had to switch over to the available local make of radiofrequency equipment for the rest of my patients since I was at a distant place from my hometown. All my surgeries done later on the substitute machine showed inferior cosmetic results with scarring. This will never occur with a scalpel.
- Improper electrical fittings and overused wires may sometimes cause shock. Electric power failure may unexpectedly occur and unless you have a generator or inverter backup, surgery will come to a standstill.

- Overused electrodes may suddenly break during surgery and unless you have a spare one you may have to work with some other configuration electrode like a triangular or diamond-shaped electrode instead of a round loop electrode, or work with a larger round loop electrode when a small-sized round loop electrode breaks. Even newer electrodes may break unexpectedly if the tissue is thick and hyperkeratotic or dry or otherwise the power used is too low and the electrode may stick in tissue and break. This spoils surgery outcome.

COMPLICATIONS DUE TO INAPPROPRIATE TECHNIQUE, LACK OF EXPERIENCE, OR OVERZEALOUS APPROACH

- Inappropriate technique and lack of experience can lead to a bigger injury due to high power or using pressure while cutting; tissue charring due to inappropriate selection of waveform (selecting electrocoagulation when electrosection or blend waveform is applicable); using a power higher than 1 when desiccating lesions, using a ball electrode for tiny lesions of verruca plana or syringoma or milia, and using the electrocoagulation waveform for such lesions on the face; using electrocoagulation for hemostasis of facial lesions. These complications can occur more commonly for newcomers and those who have shifted to radiofrequency surgery from other modalities.
- An overzealous approach is always disastrous. It can happen to experienced and inexperienced doctors who may spoil the patient's skin due to an overenthusiastic approach or under pressure from patients. This will lead to ugly scarring (Figures 18.1).

COMPLICATIONS DUE TO PATIENT'S NONCOMPLIANCE

- Patients are generally very anxious about their facial appearances and do not like downtime. Hence, facial wounds or scabs that take at least a week to improve have to be

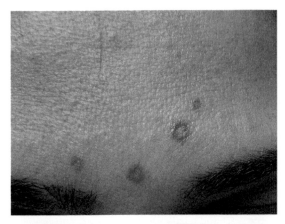
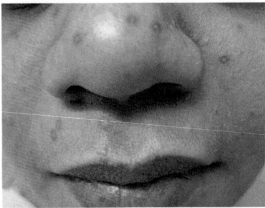

Figure 18.1 Postradiofrequency hyperpigmented scars can be caused by inappropriate settings, inexperience, or an overzealous approach.

fully understood and accepted by all patients. Any important events occurring within 8 to 15 days after procedures makes patients more anxious if the wound healing takes longer than normal time or there is sepsis. These are the situations when patients are likely to be noncompliant and use their own or some friend's ideas to improve faster instead of approaching their doctors and thus land into complications.
- Sometimes patients do not follow or complete the full course of antibiotics due to various reasons, for example, they felt better so they stopped, had side effects like rash or hyperacidity or loose motions, course of treatment was too long, or tablets or capsules were difficult to swallow.

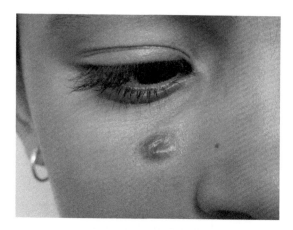

Figure 18.2 Postradiofrequency hypertrophic scar due to improper postoperative care.

- Some patients take head baths or wet the dressings often in spite of instructions or use soaps instead of the advised nonsoapy cleanser.
- Some patients move out in sunlight for long hours without the advised sun protection in spite of instructions against doing so.
- Improper follow-up visits are very common in spite of advice.
- In India, some antibiotics may be unavailable in certain areas, especially semiurban and rural areas. This leads to substitution with unmatched pharmaceutical ingredients and this may cause sepsis and scarring (Figure 18.2).
- Patients scratch and excoriate scabs or healing wounds inadvertently.
- Patients put ornaments around the neck earlier than advised.

TIPS AND TRICKS TO AVOID OR MINIMIZE COMPLICATIONS

All complications cannot be totally avoided, but with alertness, awareness, and strict protocols they can be minimized to a large extent. When complications occur, the final sufferer is the patient, but the goodwill of the doctor may also suffer as well. Next, I will enumerate and discuss ways to avoid or minimize complications.

- Always remove and wash off the surface anesthesia creams immediately after any complaints of irritation or allergy by the patient.

- Always test the local anesthetic lignocaine before surgery in spite of verbal assurance by the patient or history of previous surgery done a few weeks or months back. Before testing, the patient should have a full stomach. I always instruct patients to have food a half hour before their surgery appointment. Chances of vasovagal shock increase if the patient has an empty stomach or had food more than 3 hours before, or if the patient has come in the afternoon in hot sunlight. In case the patient has come in hot sunlight, some time should be given for him or her to settle before the test dose. Also, if the patient has eaten more than 2 hours back, I ask the patient to have a light snack or fruit juice before the test dose. Once the test is negative, the patient must sign the column in the informed consent form that mentions his or her test is negative.
- Never take a patient for surgery if the patient is too anxious or nervous, if there is vasovagal shock, or if there are symptoms and signs of allergic reaction to local anesthetic.
- The aforementioned rules apply to all ages of patients. Elderly patients have the possibility of postural hypotension, hence must be careful in handling. Extra precautions should be taken when operating on a pregnant lady (consent from her gynecologist is a must).
- Stopping of radiofrequency equipment during surgery is a once-in-a-lifetime incident. If excision is underway, one needs to complete it. This completion job may be done using a scalpel or electrocautery. If other radiofrequency equipment is available, one can use it but the parameters will never match and hence one should first try using the new equipment on wet cotton or tissue paper or a potato slice. The patient should be informed accordingly and called for follow-up more frequently. I would advise to postpone all desiccation jobs until the equipment is rectified for safety purposes.
- Have sufficient space for the equipment and wires so that there is no pull on the wires to avoid any burns or shocks. Always have a generator or inverter backup in the clinic to avoid sudden loss of power supply. The backup should be at least for 1 hour.
- Overused electrodes should be replaced with new ones on time. Disposable electrodes are always preferred. To avoid an electrode getting

stuck or entrapped in tissues, one should follow the advised optimum power for various lesions (though this varies in different machines). Electrodes should always be thoroughly cleaned as recommended after use, which maintains their good quality.

- There is no substitute for learning correct technique (refer to Chapter 8). Practice makes man perfect. There is no substitute for practice. A hasty decision to start radiofrequency surgery on a patient may lead to complications. Doctors who have switched over from other modalities surely require more practice to achieve good results.
- Any practitioner who has an overzealous approach is sure to complicate matters. Radiofrequency surgery requires fine and patient work to achieve the best results. Unrealistic expectations from patients and overpromised results from practitioners have no place in this practice. It is always best to undercorrect and achieve final results after a few weeks.
- Noncompliance from patients is a difficult area to tackle. We can only advise properly, explain everything in detail beforehand, have the informed consent signed from patients (for medicolegal consequences), and keep complete operation notes and photo documentation for all visits.

CONDITIONS TO AVOID IN OFFICE SURGERY

Finally, it is always a judicious decision of operating or not for certain lesions, which helps avoid major complications. Clinical diagnosis and a rational approach is essential in certain cases. One should also realize the limits of office dermatologic surgery. In such cases where the lesions are on sites that are vulnerable and close to certain major structures, or if the lesions are too big, or if the lesions are likely to be deep having internal connections, or with any doubtful malignant lesions, it is always a prudent decision not to operate in an office. Such lesions are on the threshold of being hospital-based operations or should be referred to a proper specialist surgeon. I am putting forth my "Say No" list for a safe office dermatologic radiofrequency surgery:

- Big-sized lesions more than 10 to 15 cm, because of problems of healing and sepsis.
- Large diffuse lesions like some lipomas, which may have deeper connections.
- Lesions on critical sites like temples, occipital areas of the scalp, near medial canthus of eyes, inside the mouth, between fingers and toes, close to external urinary meatus in males and females, inside the nostril and ear canal, in eyelashes, posterior or anterior triangles of the neck, femoral triangle, close to tortuous varicose veins, inside umbilicus, on the feet of diabetics, and very old age patients (>80 years due to possibility of compromised blood supply). A superficial epidermal lesion can be excised or desiccated in these areas safely, but deep, diffuse, and cystic lesions should be avoided in office practice.
- A protuberant swelling of unknown cause (likely malignant) that will require wide local excision or a more advanced correction method.
- Small or flat intradermal moles that will leave unsightly scars.
- Vascular lesions of large size.

19

Postradiofrequency surgery outcome

I selected radiofrequency (RF) surgery for office dermatologic surgery because of its proposed much more desirable outcome. I studied some published articles and had a firsthand experience at a clinic with a practitioner who had been using it for a couple of years. This was in 1999. The confidence of the practitioner was due to the impressive results he was able to deliver through this technology.

POSTOPERATIVE OUTCOMES

Once I started radiofrequency surgery in my office, I studied the outcome of each procedure. Outcome includes all the postoperative events until the final result. Postoperative events include all the subjective and objective experiences until the final result.

Subjective experiences

Subjective experiences after radiofrequency surgery were noted from the treated patients. I have treated more than 4000 patients with radiofrequency surgery since 1999. I have maintained a meticulous record of my cases. I typically interview my patients after surgery to get a precise opinion about the technique, its discomfort or pain, and their difficulties or problems after surgery until the present day.

I am presenting a record of 550 patients I have interviewed about their opinion on office radiofrequency surgery. Two hundred patients had excisional surgeries and 350 patients had desiccation. The details are given in Tables 19.1 and 19.2.

Table 19.1 gives the idea that after the excisional surgeries, the outcome in terms of postoperative pain and wound healing are very impressive. Patients expressed genuine satisfaction

with radiofrequency surgery and were very comfortable with the procedure.

Overall, desiccation patients expressed total satisfaction with the parameters after the procedure. The few who had problems were those who underwent treatment for numerous verruca plana, syringoma, and dermatosis papulosa nigra when they had some social embarrassment for a week after treatment because of scabs falling off late.

Objective analysis

The objective analysis of the postoperative outcome centers upon the process of wound healing, scab falling, and dyschromia and its treatment until final results.

SCAB FALLING

I have observed that the postoperative scab falling off time is directly proportional to the atmospheric humidity, that is, the higher the atmospheric humidity the longer the time the scabs will take to fall off.

Postdesiccation scab falling time is closely dependent on the following factors:

- *Atmospheric humidity*—The higher the humidity, the longer the time
- *Age of patient*—The higher the age, the longer the time
- *Size of lesion*—The larger the size, the longer the time
- *Area of treatment*—The facial area takes the least time (one week maximum), the back takes the longest (up to 15 days sometimes)
- *Sepsis*—Any sepsis or pus formation underneath will delay desquamation. The patient

Table 19.1 Opinions of 200 patients who had RF excision

Parameter	Good experience	Satisfactory experience	Poor experience
Technique	175	25	–
Postoperative pain	145 (little)	47 (some discomfort)	8 (quite painful)
Postoperative problems	158 (minor)	25 (some, especially cosmetic, had to miss work for few days)	17 (major problems of cosmetic nature for wounds on face)
Postoperative wound healing	181 (very fast)	19 (fast)	–

Table 19.2 Opinions of 350 patients who underwent RF desiccation

Parameter	Good experience	Satisfactory experience	Poor experience
Technique	312	38	None
Postoperative pain	335 (little)	15 (some discomfort)	None
Postoperative problems	296 (minor)	37 (cosmetic, especially social for facial lesions)	17 (major problems of cosmetic nature for scabs on face)
Postoperative wound healing	302 (very fast)	48 (fast)	None

may not report, as there may not be much pain. Here, during follow-up, erythema and inflammation around the scab will be noticed, or otherwise on pressure upon the scab purulent discharge will ooze out. Here, either there could be patient noncompliance or antibiotic resistant bacterial infection. Accordingly, the remedial measures have to be taken. This is most likely to lead to scarring.

Importance of automatic scab falling:

- Desiccation is always done for superficial epidermal lesions, hence scab falling will always depend upon the epidermal skin turnover or reepithelialization, which varies at different areas of the body.
- The scab normally protects the underlying wound from sepsis, hence if it prematurely falls off, the area is exposed to external infection and delayed healing as well as dyschromia and scarring.
- Premature scab falling thus also disturbs or interrupts the reepithelialization process to cause scarring.

- Superficial scabs fall off immediately within 1 to 2 days, while larger or deeper scabs take 5 to 10 days to fall off.
- Scabs on the face fall off faster than elsewhere.
- Once scabs fall off automatically, the new skin (reepithelialization) has formed. This skin will be hypopigmented or pinkish.

REEPITHELIALIZATION

- Whether excised or desiccated, the new skin appears hypopigmented and pinkish.
- This skin is thin and fragile, and can break with simple friction.
- The third phase of wound healing is collagen remodeling. This will develop new collagen tissue, which will be laid down in a systematic manner over a period of 4 to 6 weeks. The new collagen will strengthen the newly formed skin.
- The skin before the start of collagen remodeling is slightly more depressed than the original skin plane. This depression will fill up to a large extent during collagen remodeling.
- Within 2 weeks after wound healing, a phase of dyschromia sets in. Excess melanin formed

due to inflammation after the radiofrequency procedure will cause darkening of treated skin in Fitzpatrick skin types 3 to 5. Erythema will develop over the same site in Fitzpatrick skin types 1 and 2. This dyschromia settles after proper treatment in the next month.

- The treated skin finally attains its original color to blend with the adjacent normal skin 2 months after surgery. Residual dyschromia almost always clears 2 to 6 months after surgery.

FINAL RESULTS

Final results almost always appear 2 months after surgery (i.e., when the collagen remodeling phase is completed and dyschromia, if any, has settled). Results were analyzed in a subjective and objective manner. For the subjective analysis, 550 patients (200 had excisional surgeries and 350 had desiccation procedures) were interviewed about their final results (Tables 19.3 and 19.4).

The objective analysis was done separately for excisional surgeries (Figure 19.1) and desiccation procedures (Figure 19.2) with the help of photo documentation.

The final results for the excisional surgeries included the following: Atrophic scarring, especially on the face, was considered and was shallow and negligible. Dyschromia was at the end of 2 months postsurgery, which finally cleared. Hypertrophic scarring was mild and was on areas other than the face.

The final results for desiccation treatments were as follows: atrophic scarring, especially on the face, was considered, and was shallow and negligible. Dyschromia was at the end of 2 months postsurgery, which finally cleared.

Table 19.3 Response of 200 postexcision patients

	Excellent	Good	Fair	Poor
Patient responses	123	55	22	None

Table 19.4 Response of 350 postdesiccation patients

	Excellent	Good	Fair	Poor
Patient responses	270	51	29	None

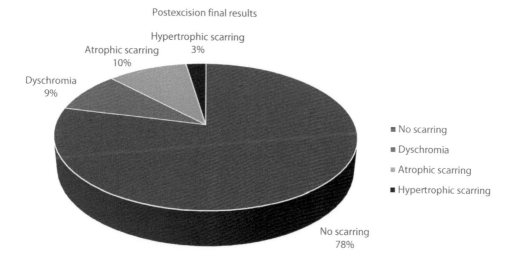

Figure 19.1 Pie chart depicting final results for excisional surgeries.

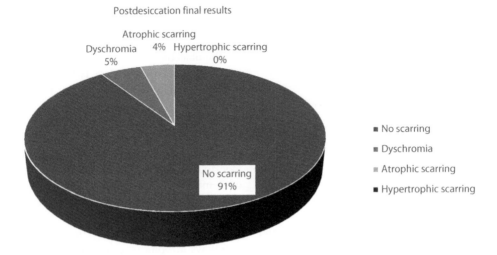

Figure 19.2 Pie chart depicting final results for desiccation treatments.

20

Achieving aesthetically superior results: Tips and tricks

Dermatologic surgery can no longer afford to be just therapeutic; it needs to also be aesthetically pleasing, because skin is nowadays more for looks than life. I mean to say that regardless of the best therapeutic result we may deliver by performing a successful dermatologic surgery, patients nowadays will demand a postsurgical result that will be aesthetically superior. Patients are against suturing, they are against a hospital stay, and against visible dressings, visible scabs, and obvious scars. They seek blemishless skin, hence they expect skin lesions to be removed without leaving any scars. They are influenced by the media which always glorifies skin, praising "flawless skin."

Patients read and express their demands directly through "straight talk." But, with our experience we need to read in between the lines and fill in the gaps left by them.

Here, I would narrate some examples from my practice. Patients ask for keloids to be removed without leaving any scars, to clear acne scars by "laser" without leaving any marks, remove any and all unsightly moles on the face or even covered areas without leaving scars, demand ear lobe repair without suturing, and many other requests. They are reluctant to have even the smallest of dressings. They have some unimaginable and fantastic ideas of anything and everything getting cleared with lasers. The word *laser* is supposed to be a magical and last word for skin lesions or blemishes, so much so that if I tell them that I will be performing their procedure with radiofrequency, they are lost and sometimes look toward me with a question mark on their faces. But, here's the scoring point for radiofrequency surgery. I will tell you how.

Radiofrequency surgery has one of the thinnest cuts in surgery, as you are aware now. In addition, it is a skillful work, which when learned gives the best and unbelievable final results so much so that our own patients become our walking and talking advertisements. Believe me, I have never really spent my money on advertising radiofrequency surgery results. Many of my walk-in patients come to me through word of mouth. This was possible because of the aesthetically superior scar after surgery and the ease of surgery in an office.

TIPS FOR AESTHETICALLY SUPERIOR RESULTS

I would like to give you some of my tips for an aesthetically superior result:

- While examining patients, always judge the depth of the lesion concerned (whether the lesion is in papillary dermis, i.e., the lesion is within 1 to 2 mm from the skin surface). This is vital as all epidermal and lesions up to the papillary dermis when removed with radiofrequency surgery are unlikely to produce scars. I say this confidently because I have experienced the very thin cut of radiofrequency surgery (10–20 microns). It cuts only the part you wish to. It will never damage the close-by skin tissue.
- Even if you are removing a deeper lesion like dermatofibroma or neurofibroma, always do blending after the excision.
- Try to remove lesions without suturing; allow secondary intention healing.

- The blending trick should be universally implemented for all lesions except those on the scalp (hairy), palms, and soles.
- Even atrophic and hypertrophic scars should be blended into surrounding skin.

TRICKS OF BLENDING TECHNIQUE

It is the blending technique that one should always master if one wishes to deliver aesthetically superior results and stand out. The blending technique remains the same for elevated or protuberant lesions and depressed lesions. The purpose of using this technique is to not only alleviate but to make the demarcation between lesions and the adjacent skin virtually invisible.

- Never use power more than 2 (this will vary from equipment to equipment).
- Always use a round loop electrode or round Surgipen.
- Always stretch the skin around the lesion slightly between the index finger and thumb of the inactive hand.
- Always keep the handpiece at an angle of 45 to 60 degrees to the skin surface plane, keep the power at 2, and do circumferential blending at the border of the removed lesion with very light or portrait-shading strokes (see Chapter 8, Figure 8.2). This procedure should be carried out over the border of the lesion (whatever may be the shape of the postoperative wound). These portrait-shading strokes will just exfoliate the stratum corneum largely to carve out and blunt the sharp border or edge.
- Later, with power at 1, keep the handpiece angulated as above or at a convenient angle (individual preference), and continue the portrait-shading of very light strokes on the adjacent normal skin to continue the blending work to actually merge the mild exfoliation done at the border into the normal skin. *There is no exfoliation done here.*
- In the aforementioned steps, the strokes are repeated at small intervals and are multiple. This procedure is always carried out under magnifying lens for best results.
- For thicker-skinned patients or when one removes a thick and hyperkeratotic lesion, power may have to be 2 for both steps.

21

Noteworthy cases

Every practitioner has interesting, unique, and noteworthy experiences to share. I believe each and every one of us have done something very different from our colleagues. It could be in the number (volume) of cases, the application of newer methods to deal with old problems, development of a simpler method to deal with the same old problems, development of a cost-effective approach, combining different techniques for a case, or developing a new application altogether. Any of these are always worth mentioning or sharing. I always believe in sharing and learning, and have been doing this at many meetings, lectures, classes, or workshops over the past 18 years of my radiofrequency surgery practice experience.

I always believe the words of Dr. Bernie Siegel: "It is always in the interest of the patient's recovery to try all kinds of promising therapies."

I will share three cases in which I feel the best features of radiofrequency surgery are worth mentioning.

CASE 1: MULTIPLE TONGUE PAPILLOMA (PAPILLOMATOSIS)

I treated this case in the early days of my practice. This patient was carrying these multiple warts over his tongue for a year (Figure 21.1), and had consulted various doctors (general surgeon, oto-rhinolaryngologist, dermatologist, faciomaxillary surgeon, and homeopathic and Ayurvedic specialists). He was treated with electrocautery and excision, which were followed by recurrence. The patient was himself a radiologist.

How I treated this case:

- I asked the patient to use a lignocaine viscous solution for topical anesthesia before coming to the clinic. This gave a sufficient numbing effect. In case the numbing was not up to the desired level, I injected lignocaine 2% underneath the warty lesions.
- I used a broad needle electrode. Power was 2 to 4 maximum. The waveform selected was electrodessication.
- The lesions were touched for 5 to 10 seconds at intervals of half a minute several times until the warts showed visible whitening due to dehydration or a bit of charring by the browning effect on warty tissue.
- These lesions were then left to desquamate and fall off automatically. This happened in a week's time.
- The patient was treated fortnightly four to five times. This cleared all warts completely.
- Follow-up was done fortnightly for 3 months for recurrence.
- Any recurrences were immediately treated.
- There were no other features of immunodeficiency.
- There has been no recurrence in the past 15 years and the result is excellent to date.

Postprocedure pain was bearable and lasted for the whole day of the procedure. The treated lesions desquamated within one week each time. Recurrence is less because in electrodessication, the electrocoagulation waveform is used and the heat generated dissipates into surrounding tongue tissue deeper to

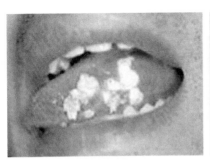
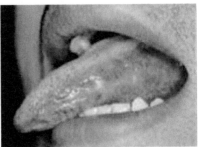

Figure 21.1 Multiple warts on left side of tongue cleared completely with no recurrence. (From Biju Vasudevan, *Procedural Dermatosurgery, A Step by Step Approach*, Jaypee Brothers Medical Book Publishers Pvt. Ltd., 2018.)

cause necrosis at least a millimeter away from the lesion thus clearing off the newly invaded cells.

Take-home message: The electrodessication technique used judiciously and convincingly has the potential to deliver marvelous results. It may take a longer time to give a complete result but it is less painful, more acceptable, and more convincing. It scores over all other modalities and is definitely far better than surgical excision done by an otorhinolaryngologist, or oral or general surgeon.

CASE 2: GIANT CONDYLOMA ACUMINATA ON PERIANAL AREA

This was a case of an 18-year-old male patient, who I treated two years back. He had consulted general practitioners and specialists near his native place outside India and was offered some treatment that did not help. He had come for a vacation to India where his grandparents lived. When I saw him he had huge masses of warty tissue (florid appearance) growing at the perianal area near the anal orifice. He had approached me for complaints of bleeding per rectum. He had developed sepsis in those masses and was foul smelling. He was treated with liquid podophyllum 2 days earlier by a dermatologist. I treated him with an oral antibiotic and called for review after 2 days. On the follow-up visit I started photo documentation and advised radiofrequency treatment in two to three sessions at 1- to 2-week intervals (Figures 21.1 to 21.9).

How I treated this case:

- This patient was treated in the operation theater of a hospital on a daycare basis.
- Lidocaine 15% w/w topical aerosol was sprayed on the warts a few minutes before giving

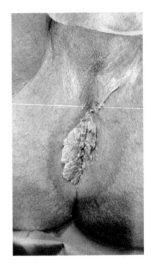

Figure 21.2 Giant condyloma acuminata on perianal area.

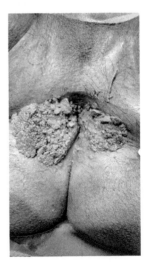

Figure 21.3 Giant condyloma acuminata on perianal area.

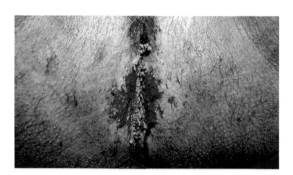

Figure 21.4 Immediately after first session of treatment (blood oozing).

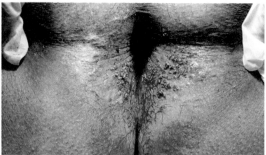

Figure 21.7 Immediately after second session.

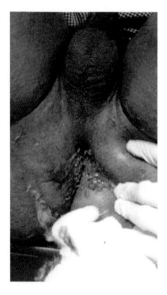

Figure 21.5 One week after first session.

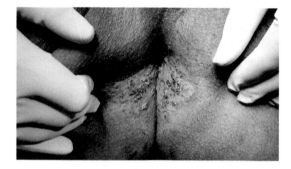

Figure 21.8 One week after second session.

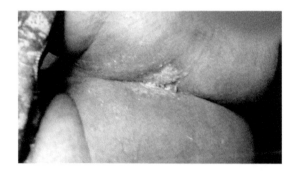

Figure 21.6 Two weeks after first session.

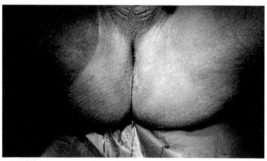

Figure 21.9 One month after second session.

- A broad needle electrode was used at a power of 2 to 4.
- The electrode vaporized all the superficial warts very fast.
- The significant smoke generated was evacuated with powerful exhaust fans.
- The necrosed tissues were cleared by wiping with normal saline solution.
- Capillary bleeding emerged from the wounds, which stopped with pressure at some places.

injectable lignocaine 2% with adrenaline underneath the warty tissue.
- Electrosection or the cut waveform was selected to treat lesions for its very fine tissue destruction or its use in radiovaporization.

- Other bleeding areas were electrocoagulated as usual.
- The wounds were dressed with povidone iodine ointment and the dressing changed daily after defecation.
- Normal saline was advised for daily cleaning of wounds.
- Broad spectrum oral antibiotic Cefuroxime Axetil 500 mg twice daily was given for one week. For pain relief Ibuprofen 400 mg thrice daily was advised for 2 to 3 days.
- Patient was followed up after one week and 50% of the lesions showed clearing.
- The second session was followed on similar lines after 3 weeks, which cleared all the warty remnants fully.
- Per-rectal examination was done using a speculum to find out if any warts were present inside the anal canal or rectum. Examination revealed no such growths.
- Patient recovered completely without recurrence until today.

Postprocedure pain was bearable and there were no complications or sepsis. The postoperative period was uneventful and smooth.

Take-home message: These giant or large sized lesions were treated using the gem of radiovaporization, which helped vaporize all warts very fast in just two sessions within a span of one month. Expert general surgeons and plastic surgeons who were consulted for a second opinion had planned wide local excision followed by a flap to heal the large wound. Radiofrequency surgery wins over in such cases.

CASE 3: POSTTRAUMATIC PUNCHED OUT SCAR ON TIP OF NOSE

This case was a postaccidental scar on the nose tip of a 25-year-old male. This patient had developed a deep punched out scar of about 1 cm diameter of 6 months duration. I treated this case 15 years ago. I used the pearl technique of radiofrequency resurfacing to improve the scar in a single session (Figure 21.10).

How I treated this case:

- Lignocaine 2% with adrenaline was injected underneath the scar.
- The scar was resurfaced with a round Surgipen electrode.
- The cut waveform was selected.
- Power adjustments and the three steps technique was the same described in chapter.
- The postprocedure wound was like a superficial abrasion.
- The wound healed with secondary intention.
- Postoperative care and advice remain the same as described earlier.
- Postprocedure dyschromia (hyperpigmentation) developed 4 weeks following treatment. It was cleared with bleaching creams within 1 month.
- Scar depth improved to the extent of 60% of the original with the new collagen formation and very good blunting of edges.

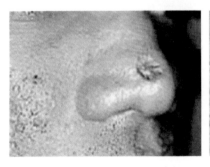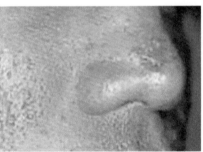

Figure 21.10 Posttraumatic punched out scar on tip of nose shows excellent resurfacing in single session. (From Biju Vasudevan, *Procedural Dermatosurgery, A Step by Step Approach*, Jaypee Brothers Medical Book Publishers Pvt. Ltd., 2018.)

- After 2 months I treated the same scar with a 50% glycolic acid solution-based chemical peel, especially at the edge to further flatten them (spot peel).
- This helped the same scar to show a great improvement in the next 2 months.

This scar was a real challenge to resurface (or revise). First, the location on the tip of the nose was itself a crucial one where the flesh or soft tissue was not present to lay down the "lift-up grip." The postoperative pain was bearable and healing was as expected.

Take-home message: It is possible to resurface deep punched out scars to the extent of 50% to 60% in a single session with the unique method described in Chapter 15. This is a very skillful method and does not require prior subcision. Subcision, if done, will surely give an enhanced result. Proper scar selection is essential for the best result, which can be equivalent or even better than laser resurfacing or punch excision and grafting.

22

From fantasy to factuality

I took the one less traveled by, And that has made all the difference.

Robert Frost

The great Albert Einstein once said, "Imagination is more important than knowledge." I always believe this statement has a great meaning. Only having knowledge will be in vain if there are no ideas or innovative thinking to create new uses.

The right brain has qualities of imagination and creativity, whereas the left brain has qualities of intelligence and knowledge. For innovative thinking, a harmonious coordination and synergy of both brains is required. (See Figure 22.1.)

Here I remember one quotation that was displayed outside the pathology specimen hall at B. J. Medical College that said, "To know is not only to know, but to know and to doubt, hence not to know everything." I liked it so much that it has become my inspiring thought all these years.

Henry Thoreau once said, "A good question is never answered. It is not a bolt to be tightened into place, but a seed to be planted and to bear more seeds toward the hope of greening the landscape of ideas." Nothing in the world is as great as an idea.

A dermatologic surgeon too must have "fantasy" in order to be successful. But he or she should make the best use of pathological knowledge to plan and execute the "factual" elements. Using the best of today's technology he or she can develop innovative methods to generate new applications or improvise older methods.

A patient's fantasy is many times unimaginable. Some young males and females try to copy their most favorite film stars and come with some fantastic demands that can never be fulfilled. For example, some ladies request that all the moles on their face be removed. They have the impression that they can have "a clean skin" (clean and clear skin). They are misguided either by media or friends. They are of firm belief that they can have clean and clear skin by using a laser just the same way how they can have a hairless body with laser. They see any and all small pigmented macules as unwanted defects on their facial skin that should be removed without leaving any blemishes. They see any and all tiny depressions on the facial skin as scars and demand removal.

This patient fantasy can be turned into a reality with the help of factuality, which can be explained with the help of science and technology. Patients need to be made to understand the difference in the morphology of the particular pigmented macules and their feasibility to best treatment without leaving scars.

Modern-day technological advancements have seen the development of high-power lasers (large variety), radiofrequency, and ultrasound. Out of these, lasers have become the most sought after technology by medical professionals. Huge sums of money have been pumped into developing new lasers (ablative, nonablative, fractionated, ultrapulsed, superpulsed, nanosecond, picosecond, dual wavelength, and many more). Newer lasers keep hitting the market with huge investments by medical professionals for improving their own results

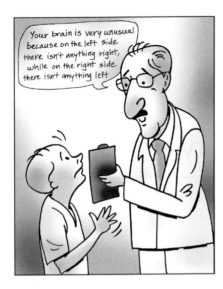

Figure 22.1 In lighter vein.

the most important subjects are laser–tissue interactions and laser physics.

When doing dermatologic surgery using modalities other than the scalpel, three effects are most important:

1. Vaporization (cellular and extracellular water evaporation and boiling)
2. Coagulation (blood clotting, protein denaturation)
3. Carbonization (tissue charring)

The first and second are desired and utilized in dermatologic surgery. This is adequately covered in earlier chapters. Radiofrequency surgery has its clear advantages in the aforementioned effects as you know now. Hence, I consider radiofrequency surgery a refinement in dermatologic and aesthetic surgery. It holds the following advantages not only over other modalities, as discussed earlier, but scores over lasers due to the following characteristics:

- Small, portable equipment
- Very affordable
- Very versatile (many applications with single equipment)
- No more modifications or updating
- Low maintenance costs
- Consumes much less power, easily works on simple inverters in case of power failures
- Single electrode can last for dozens of procedures
- Color-blind, hence can treat many disorders or lesions
- No fixed parameters or protocols (case individuality)
- No lengthy learning curve
- Therapeutic and diagnostic (biopsy possible) value

Last, I would like to enumerate once again the many benefits of radiofrequency surgery for dermatologic surgery:

- Absolutely precise incision
- Pressureless incision
- Least lateral tissue thermal damage, hence least charring
- Very fine cut as though tissue is just "split" or "divided" by touch

(quality-wise) and reducing side effects, thus offering patients the "latest and most advanced" every few years for the same indications. There is also a plethora of presentations and publications from company-sponsored workshops or actual unbiased clinical experiences from the medical professionals globally trying to prove how the latest technology is better than the previous one. There is no doubt that lasers are perhaps the most amazing achievements of our time and enjoy a wide array of indications in the field of medicine, but at the same time medical professionals need to understand the basics that lasers are color sensitive (wavelength-specific color absorption) and hence if used blindly can damage the skin irreparably.

Lasers have amazing precision and the programs are computer based. These programs may be tailor-made for certain indications but they have to be modified to suit the skin of color and the lesion in focus. This is pure science and has to be applied from case to case. Hence, lasers cannot be considered a universal remedy by any medical professional. A single laser can never treat vast indications. For that medical professionals need to have either a range of lasers or a platform having different heads used for different indications. The cost for such investment is phenomenal, plus the ever-changing research and technology bringing newer models every year. I have seen few patients being spoiled by using a single laser for many unindicated lesions or using higher-than-indicated energy. Lasers have a longer learning curve where

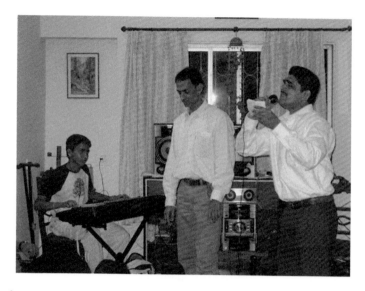

Figure 22.2 Radiofrequency surgery is like a keyboard: versatile.

- Almost bloodless operative field due to simultaneous hemostasis
- Incision always sterile
- Easy modifications of power and waveform to suit the applications
- Very clean postoperative wounds
- Postoperative pain or discomfort is far less
- Fast postoperative healing
- Minimal postoperative complications
- Soft or negligible postoperative scarring
- Versatility of applications
- Superior results

With radiofrequency surgery, the art of dermatologic surgery to give superior aesthetic results is very much possible making best use of the scientific knowledge of this technique. Finally, it is the patient who judges the result he or she experiences. It is the patients themselves who have recommended or endorsed radiofrequency surgery as their choice.

In a concert or orchestra, if you have a keyboard player, you do not have to depend upon availability of other musicians for performance, as the keyboard is a versatile musical equipment (Figure 22.2). Similarly, in dermatologic surgery if you have radiofrequency surgery equipment and have mastered its use, you are miles ahead of your colleagues when it comes to dermatologic surgery.

Experience tells you what to do; confidence allows you to do it.

Stan Smith

Index

Page numbers followed by f and t indicate figures and tables, respectively.

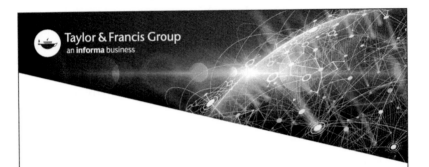

Printed and bound by CPI Group (UK) Ltd, Croydon, CR0 4YY

24/10/2024

01778290-0017